A Handbook of Oral Physiology and Oral Biology

By

Anastasios K. Markopoulos, DDS, MS, PhD

Professor of Oral Medicine/Pathology, Aristotle University,
Thessaloniki, Greece

CONTENTS

FOREWORD

Oral biology deals with the biochemical, chemical, molecular biologic, general biologic and physical aspects of all processes that take place in the oral cavity, in the masticatory organ, and in the associated tissues and body fluids. From the methodological point of view, oral biology is indistinguishable from basic sciences.

In this book, Professor Markopoulos excellently discusses the fundamental aspects of the structure and function of the oral mucosal cells and its specializations, which allow oral mucosa to fulfill several roles. He successfully also covers other important topics, such as aspects of bone biology, oral microbiology, mastication, deglutition and speech.

Antonis Konstantinidis, DDS, MSc, PhD

Professor & Chairman of Preventive Dentistry, Periodontology and Implant Biology
School of Dentistry, Aristotle University, Thessaloniki, Greece

PREFACE

Oral Biology is concerned with the nature of the oral and craniofacial tissues and with the application of basic scientific knowledge to oral tissues in health and disease. Oral Biology is a tremendously diverse scientific area, encompassing the disciplines of molecular biology and genetics, microbiology and immunology, biochemistry, biophysics, craniofacial biology and development, pharmacology and physiology. The aim of the present book is to illustrate how fundamental biologic phenomena are involved in the oral diseases. I've tried to produce a book, which provides a comprehensive brief overview of the entire field of oral biology and oral physiology. I hope that the book will be of value not only to under- and graduate students, but also to dental practitioners. It will have served a useful purpose if it poses more questions than it answers.

Anastasios K.Markopoulos, DDS, MS, PhD
Professor of Oral Medicine/Pathology
Aristotle University, Thessaloniki, Greece

CHAPTER 1

Structure and Function of the Cells of Oral Mucosa

Anastasios K. Markopoulos

Aristotle University of Thessaloniki

Abstract: The mucosa lining the oral cavity varies significantly in its structure and function. In some areas of the mouth, it protects the underlying structures; in others, it provides a means of transepithelial absorption and around the teeth it provides a unique epithelial structure and controls passage of crevicular fluid. This chapter reviews briefly the major structural characteristics of the cells of oral epithelium and connective tissue. The elementary cell mechanisms and functions of keratinocytes and every cell of the connective tissue are also briefly analyzed.

STRUCTURE AND FUNCTION OF ORAL EPITHELIAL CELLS

The typical cell consists of cytoplasm and a nucleus, which is surrounded by a double-layered porous nuclear membrane. Nucleus contains the genetic material and controls all the cell's functions.

Nucleolus is a non-membrane bound structure composed of proteins and nucleic acids found within the nucleus. It contains RNA and is considered the site of mRNA, rRNA and tRNA synthesis.

Cytoplasm surrounds the nucleus and contains several organelles, such as, endoplasmic reticulum, ribosomes, Golgi apparatus, lysosomes, peroxisomes, mitochondria, centrosomes and cytoskeleton.

Endoplasmic reticulum is subdivided in the rough and smooth reticulum. Rough endoplasmic reticulum participates in the synthesis of proteins that are used or excreted by the cell. Smooth endoplasmic reticulum lacks ribosomes and contributes to the synthesis of glycoprotein carbohydrates.

Ribosomes Constitute the Sites of Protein Synthesis

Golgi apparatus participates in the transportation of proteins through the endoplasmic reticulum. Transportation is mainly achieved with the help of excretory vesicles, which attach and coalesce to the cell membrane.

Lysosomes contain hydrolytic enzymes that have the capability to digest old organelles, bacteria, fungi and viruses.

Peroxisomes mainly contain peroxidases and catalases. Their role is significant in the metabolic processes and in the inactivation of various toxic products.

Mitochondria are oval-shaped formations surrounded by double membrane. They represent the site of ATP synthesis that provides energy to the cell.

Centrosomes are a pair of centrioles mainly consisting of microtubules and participating in the cell division.

Cytoskeleton consists of microtubules, intermediate fibrils and microfibrils.

Microtubules are tubular formations 25nm in diameter. They are found in centrioles and on the cell projections (flagellae).

Intermediate fibrils consist of a three fibrils network, 10 nm in total diameter. They are interconnected with ribosomes, mitochondria and other cell organelles.

Microfibrils are also tubular formations, 7 nm in diameter. They participate in the mitotic activity.

Cellular projections are found in the exterior surface of cell and are subdivided in microvilli, in cilia and in flagellae.

Microvilli) project from the surface of cells and are usually found in the epithelial cells. Cilia are structures resembling hairs and are located on the surface of respiratory epithelium cells. Flagellae are mainly found in sperm cells.

Cell membrane represents a separating limit between the intracellular and extracellular environment. A double layer of proteins and lipids presenting hydrophobic and hydrophilic regions constitutes it.

The main components of cellular membrane are phospholipids, cholesterol, various glycoproteins and glycolipids.

Movement and transportation of proteins and glycoproteins takes place inside the cell membrane, while the movement of phospholipids can be performed inside and outside the membrane (model of "humid mosaic" for the cellular membranes).

The basic operations of cell membranes are the maintenance of integrity of the cell, the mechanical support of its shape, and the facilitation of passage of water-soluble molecules. They also constitute the site of various hormonal receptors, they regulate metabolic processes (with enzymatic help) and they have the ability to recognize other cells.

Transportation of Derivatives in and Outside the Cell

This process is performed with simple or facilitated diffusion, with osmosis and with energetic transportation.

Simple diffusion is a passive phenomenon and is based on the movement of the dissolved substance from a bigger to a lower concentration.

Facilitated diffusion is the spontaneous passage of molecules or ions across a biological membrane. Facilitated diffusion is a passive phenomenon. The transporter is specific transmembrane proteins of cellular membrane. Example of facilitated diffusion is the transport of glucose in the cell.

Osmosis is a phenomenon, characterized by diffusion of water via a selectively permeable membrane. The movement of water takes place from the higher to the lower concentration.

For the process of energetic transportation, ATP is used. In energetic transportation, the movement from low in higher concentration is possible. Example of energetic transportation is Na^+/K^+ pump.

Endocytosis

Endocytosis is carried out with three ways: with phagocytosis, pinocytosis and endocytosis via the cellular membrane.

Phagocytosis is an energetic phenomenon, which aims at the destruction of cells or bacteria.

Pinocytosis is an energetic phenomenon that aims at the uptake by the cell of external liquid or dissolved substances.

Endocytosis via the cellular membrane aims at the uptake of special molecules. For this purpose, the receptors of cellular membrane encounter the special molecules. Example of endocytosis via the cellular membrane is the uptake of hormones in cells-targets [1].

Exocytosis

Exocytosis is the extrusion of useless substances from the cell. The useless substances are encompassed from specific vesicles, which coalesce with the cellular membrane for the extrusion of the substance.

In cases where the extruded substance is useful for the organism, the term excretion is used instead.

Reproduction of Epithelial Cells

Cellular division is continuous and aims at the renewal of cells. The number of new cells is equal with the number of apoptotic cells. Cellular division occurs in the upper basal layer of epithelium. In the epithelium of attached gingiva, cellular division is carried out near the epithelial rete ridges. The intensity of cellular division is higher in the non-keratinized epithelium. Mitotic index is the percentage of dividing cells in a certain unit of time.

The cell cycle consists of four distinct phases: G_1 phase, S phase (synthesis), G_2 phase (collectively known as interphase) and M phase (mitosis). M phase is itself composed of two tightly coupled processes: mitosis, in which the cell's chromosomes are divided between the two daughter cells, and cytokinesis, in which the cell's cytoplasm divides, forming distinct cells.

Mitosis is subdivided into several distinct phases, sequentially known as prophase, prometaphase, metaphase, anaphase and telophase.

PHASES OF CELLULAR CYCLE

G1 is considered phase of rest of the cell. Between mitotic (m) and G1 phase the cell "takes" the decision if it will remain in the ancestral form or it will be differentiated in order to reach in the upper layers of epithelium.

S phase is characterized by DNA synthesis that is required for the cellular division. G2 phase is considered premitotic phase with no visible histologic findings. In the initial stages of M phase (prophase and metaphase) chromosome formation and presence of mitotic spindle are apparent. In anaphase and telophasis removal of chromosomes and diametrical presence of chromosomes are evident. Finally, in cytokinesis the maternal cell splits in two daughter cells that each one has the same number of chromosomes as the maternal cell (46 chromosomes).

Aim of mitosis is growth and repair.

The time duration of mitotic phase varies from 30-60 min. G1 phase lasts from 14-140 h while S and G2 phase from 9 -11 h.

Functions of Epithelial Cells

The epithelium of the oral mucosa is constituted by two major categories of cells; keratinocytes and non-keratinocytes.

Keratinocytes originate from the basal layer of epithelium and their mission is to ascend in the upper layers of epithelium in order to undergo keratinization.

Non-keratinocytes include four types of cells, melanocytes, Langerhans cells, Merkel cells and lymphocytes. Melanocytes originate from neural crest and their functional mission is the production of melanin.

Langerhans cells originate from bone marrow. They are considered the most peripheral organs of the immune system participating in the immune reactions of the oral mucosa and presenting antigens to T lymphocytes.

Merkel cells originate from neural crest. Their probable function is the participation in sensory functions of the oral mucosa (mainly with the touch).

BASEMENT MEMBRANE

The basement membrane is a thin continuous zone with which the epithelium joins with connective tissue. It follows a wave-like course proportional with the epithelial rete ridges. The basement membrane becomes visible with PAS or silver stainings. It has a thickness of 1-2 mm and is constituted by four regions: a) the cellular membrane of the cells of basal layer of epithelium b) clear zones (lamina lucida) c) the dark area (lamina densa) and d) the reticular layer.

In reality it is not a membrane; it is a complex of fibrils, which interlock collagen fibrils of the connective tissue with lamina densa and lamina lucida and with the epithelium.

The cellular membrane of basal cells of epithelium has hemidesmosomes, from which integrins and anchor collagen fibrils depart, leading to the dark area and reticular layer respectively. A network, formed by anchor collagen fibrils (collagen of type VII) and collagen fibers of type I and III that are secreted by fibroblasts constitutes the reticular layer.

The basal membrane is considered a molecular filter allowing the permeability of nutritious substances from connective tissue to epithelium, since the epithelium is deprived of vessels. It also influences cellular differentiation and proliferation.

STRUCTURE AND FUNCTION OF CELLS OF THE CONNECTIVE TISSUE

The connective tissue is composed of ground substance, fibers and cells.

The ground substance is mainly constituted of carbohydrate-protein complexes.

The fibers of connective tissue are composed of collagen, reticular, elastic fibers and oxytalan fibers.

The cells of connective tissue are the fibroblasts, histiocytes, macrophages, polymorphonuclear cells, lymphocytes and mast cells.

Functions of Fibroblasts

The basic mission of fibroblasts is the production of fibers and ground substance.

Functions of Polymorphonuclear Cells

Polymorphonuclear cells are cells with phafocytic capabilities and play important role in the acute phase of inflammation. In order to perform their phagocytic action they participate in several complex operations. Initially, they are attached in the wall of vessel and afterwards they migrate at the site of inflammation via the phenomena of migration and chemotaxis. Then they are exposed to the bacterium or the foreign body. The contact is usually performed with the help of cell membrane receptors for IgG or C3 that polymorphonuclear cells possess. Cell membrane surrounds the bacterium, a phagosome is formed, and inside the phagosome, enzymes are released that dissolve the intruder.

Functions of Histiocytes - Macrophages

Histiocytes are considered progenitor form of macrophages.

Macrophages play an important role in the defense against various microbial factors. Macrophages that carry out this activity may be "physiological" or activated.

Macrophages contribute in:

1. Defense against microorganisms

2. Excretion of dead cells and useless substances

3. Regulatory action in hematopoiesis

4. Synthesis of biologically active substances

5. They also participate in the immune reactions (presentation of antigens to lymphocytes)

Macrophages have the ability of interferon production. They also help lymphocytes for interferon production.

Functions of Lymphocytes

Central lymphatic organs differentiate and activate lymphocytes. The role of thymus is to differentiate the lymphocytes that pass from this gland, in immunocompetent T lymphocytes. In bone marrow, differentiation of lymphocytes to B cells takes place.

After their activation T lymphocytes enter in the blood circulation (lymph nodes-thoracic duct-blood). In the lymph nodes, T lymphocytes reside in the cortex, in the so-called thymus-dependent regions. Some of the mature T lymphocytes migrate from blood to the spleen or even to bone marrow, where they can survive up to 20 years. This fact explains why the inactivity of thymus in adults does not significantly influence cellular immunity. T lymphocytes are related with the cellular part of immunity.

B lymphocytes are produced in bone marrow. Later they migrate via the blood circulation in the peripheral lymphatic organs, where accepting antigenic irritations are differentiated to plasma cells. Plasma cells produce the antibodies. B cells are found in abundance in the germ centers of lymph nodes and in the diffuse lymphatic tissue (tonsils, appendix and Peyer patches). They are also found in small numbers in the blood in the form of inactive or rested lymphocytes. B lymphocytes participate in the humoral part of immunity.

Functions of Eosinophils

Usually they are found in inflammatory conditions. Their phagocytic ability is smaller compared with polymorphonuclear cells. They are believed to produce cationic granule proteins, reactive oxygen species such as superoxide, lipid mediators like the eicosanoids and prostaglandins, enzymes, growth factors (TGF, VEGF, and PDGF) and cytokines such as IL-1, IL-2, IL-4, IL-5, IL-6, IL-8, IL-13, and TNF alpha. They also play a role in fighting viral infections Eosinophils along with basophils and mast cells, are important mediators of allergic responses. Eosinophils are also involved in allograft rejection and neoplasia. They have also recently been implicated in antigen presentation to T cells [2-8].

Functions of Basophils and Mast Cells

Basophils are smaller in size cells of the white line. Their cytoplasm contains quantities of histamine and heparin. Their role in phagocytosis is limited. They have active participation in the allergic reactions.

Mast cells contain heparin and histamine, substances affecting the coagulation of blood, the vessels and the smooth muscular fibers. The role of mast cells is significant in type I anaphylactic reactions.

REFERENCES

[1]   Doherty GJ, McMahon HT. Mechanisms of endocytosis. Biochemistry 2009; 78:857-902.

[2]   Bandeira-Melo C, Bozza P, Weller P. The cellular biology of eosinophil eicosanoid formation and function. J Allergy Clin Immunol 2002; 109: 393–400.

[3]   Horiuchi T, Weller P. Expression of vascular endothelial growth factor by human eosinophils: upregulation by granulocyte macrophage colony-stimulating factor and interleukin-5. Am J Respir Cell Mol Biol 1997; 17: 70–7.

[4]   Kato Y, Fujisawa T, Nishimori H, *et al*. Leukotriene D4 induces production of transforming growth factor-beta1 by eosinophils. Int Arch Allergy Immunol 2005; 137 (Suppl 1): 17–20.

[5]   Rothenberg M, Hogan S. The eosinophil. Ann Rev Immunol 2006; 24: 147–74.

[6]   Saito K, Nagata M, Kikuchi I, Sakamoto Y. Leukotriene D4 and eosinophil transendothelial migration, superoxide generation, and degranulation via beta2 integrin. Ann Allergy Asthma Immunol 2004; 93: 594–600.

[7]   Shi H. Eosinophils function as antigen-presenting cells. J Leukoc Biol 2004; 76:520-7.

[8]   Trulson A, Byström J, Engström A, Larsson R, Venge P. The functional heterogeneity of eosinophil cationic protein is determined by a gene polymorphism and post-translational modifications. Clin Exp Allergy 2007; 37: 208–18.

CHAPTER 2

Biology of Bone

Anastasios K. Markopoulos

Aristotle University of Thessaloniki

Abstract: Bones are rigid organs that form part of the endoskeleton of vertebrates. They function to move, support, and protect the various organs of the body, produce <u>red</u> and white blood cells and store minerals. This chapter briefly covers a wide spectrum of areas related to elementary bone pathophysiological features and basic bone research. While bone embryology, osteogenesis, bone remodeling, bone development, osteoblast and osteoclast biology constitute the main contents, topics important to the understanding of bone metabolic diseases are also reviewed. The significance of bone enhancing factors and effect of immune system on bone is discussed. Elementary knowledge is also given for the relation of bone and implants.

THE BONE AS AN ORGAN

Bone can be considered as a tissue and as an organ. Bone is a major supporting tissue. It is very similar to other connective tissues. It is considered supportive calcified tissue [1].

It is also part of an organ system. It has to do with movement and protection. Bone is a storehouse of minerals. It also has to do with protection of the brain and spinal cord.

Totally, human skeleton has 206 bones.

According to their shape, bones are distinguished in:

- ✓ long bones
- ✓ short bones
- ✓ flat bones and
- ✓ irregular bones

In gross sections of bone, we see:

- ✓ compact bone (cortical)
- ✓ cancellous bone (spongeous)

These two types of bone constitute all bones. On the surface of joints, there is subchondral tissue. This forms underneath cartilage. It has numerous blood vessels to carry blood to cartilage.

Cartilage has no blood vessels. Any bone microscopically has the same picture. Adult bone is called lamellar bone.

Bone is a highly metabolic unit involved in a big number of functions (osteogenic, hemopoetic).

Regardless from how bone is embryologically formed, its final picture in all cases ends up the same.

From embryologic point of view, bone can derive from

- ✓ intramembranous or
- ✓ endochondreal osteogenesis

Early bone is named embryonic, primary, or woven bone.

On the contrary, mature bone called adult, secondary, or lamellar bone.

Primary and secondary bone can co-exist in certain regions of skeleton (cranial bones).

EMBRYOLOGY OF BONE

Embryogenesis of bone may be: (I) intramembranous and (II) endochondreal.

INTRAMEMBRANOUS OSTEOGENESIS

Although ovulation and fertilization do not coincide chronologically, they are considered as day one in the embryonic life.

After the stage of fertilization, cells are moved and are implanted in the endometrium of uterus. This process requires approximately 11-12 days. During this movement, we have cell division (stage of zygote).

After this stage, we have the formation of morula, which consists of 64 or more cells (stage of morula).

As division goes on in the morula, a space begins to form amongst those cells. This space is named blastocyst (stage of blastocyst).

As cellular division continues, the formation of inner cell mass takes place. The inner cell mass mounts the blastocyst on the endometrium (stage of implantation). The inner cell mass continues to grow. Then, we have the beginning of the three primary layers; the ectoderm, the endoderm and the mesoderm. Bone and cartilage originate from mesoderm.

As the neural tube grows, neural crest is formed. After its formation, it migrates into the tissues of the embryo where several different things shown below are formed:

- ✓ cranial sensory ganglion cells
- ✓ posterior root ganglion cells
- ✓ Schwann cells
- ✓ autonomic ganglion cells
- ✓ supradrenal medulla cells
- ✓ melanocytes

Why neural crest is important? Because all mesenchymal tissues of the head and neck are derived from neural crest. All connective tissues of the head and neck are derived from the ectodermal tissue of the neural tube. Their name is ectomesenchyme. In the rest body from head and down, bone is derived from mesoderm.

Formation of somites from mesoderm also takes place in the whole body, except from head and neck region where formation stops.

At the fifth week of embryonal life compensation and differentiation of cells occurs.

The differentiation of cells depends on two important factors:

- ✓ internal genome
- ✓ environmental factors (which helps the genome to be expressed)

At the seventh week, some of these differentiated cells have become cartilaginous.

At the eighth week, we have:

- ✓ abundance of cartilage
- ✓ beginning of calcification (bone formation)

Where intramembranous ossification takes place?

- ✓ in the frontal bone of skull and
- ✓ in other bones of cranial bowl
- ✓ in the maxilla
- ✓ in the mandible

The other bones of skeleton are calcified endochondreally. Generally, in any bone under the periosteum, osteogenesis is intramembranous. At the 8th week, we have the formation of primary ossification centers in the bones of cranial bones (first in the frontal bone). The formation process starts with compensation of mesenchymal cells. Then mesenchymal cells differentiate to osteoprogenitor cells, which in turn differentiate to osteoblasts.

Diagrammatically: Mesenchymal cells → Differentiation of mesenchymal cells→ Osteoprogenitor cells → Differentiation of osteoprogenitor cells → osteoblasts

Mesenchymal cells　　　　=　stem cells

Osteoprogenitor cells　　=　osteoprogenitor or intermediate cells

Osteoblasts　　　　　　　=　Cells in the end of differentiation

The same process occurs in endochondreal bone formation.

After this stage of primary ossification centers formation, osteoblasts take a spheroidal membrane form and begin to secrete some products inside the surface of the sphere.

- ✓ collagen
- ✓ non-collagenous proteins
- ✓ matrix vesicles and
- ✓ glycosoaminoglucans

Matrix vesicles are the initial sites of calcification. They cannot easily be identified in the light microscope because they are too small. Inside and around matrix vesicles, hydroxyapatite crystals are growing and form bone nodules (woven bone).

Characteristics of the woven bone are:

- ✓ no distinct orientation of collagen (it is formed rapidly)
- ✓ nodular substructure

Afterwards, osteoblasts stop secreting matrix vesicles and start secreting oriented collagen. The signal for this change, which finally leads to development of lamellar bone, is given from the genome of these osteoblasts. There is no external signal. Later, multinucleated cells (osteoclasts) appear. As bone is formed, it is reabsorbed by osteoclasts.

ENDOCHONDREAL OSTEOGENESIS

At the 5th week of uterine life, we see compensation of mesenchymal cells. At the 7th week, these cells differentiate into cartilage precursors. The steps in endochondreal bone formation are the same as in intramembranous. The difference is that in intramembranous we have bone formation directly in the mesenchymal connective tissue, while in endochondreal bone formation in the specules of cartilage that have been destroyed. If we go to the fetal week, we observe some bone formation taking place. For the first formation of bone, we see some primary ossification centers in the middle of the bone (diaphesis). In every long bone, there is one ossification center. In this area, there is condensed mesenchyma and cartilage precursors are found. These cells produce a different kind of extracellular matrix. The characteristics of cartilage are the abundant presence of chondroitin sulphate and the presence of cells that are residing in some spaces called lacunae. We can also see differentiation of mesenchymal cells into a fibrous coverage of cartilage. This fibrous cover is named perichondrium. Perichondrium has two layers; an outer, which is the fibrous part, and an inner, which is the chondrogenic layer. The growth of cartilage takes place with two ways; appositionaly (more and more matrix) and interstitialy (from the chondrogenic part). Cartilage matrix is producing collagen, which is very fine and not very well polymerized. This is type II collagen. As blood vessels grow in the external part of cartilage, they cause changes in its microenvironment and initiate differentiation of the perichondreal cells (of the chondrogenic layer) into osteoprogenitor cells and osteoblasts.

Interestingly, because perichondreal cells have differentiated from the fibrous layer and produce bone not because of cartilage being their first, the produced bone is intramembranous. A general rule therefore is that periosteal bone is always intramembranous.

The steps in the endochondreal bone formation are:

✓ Periosteum formation

✓ Due to lack of vascularization or due to calcification of matrix, the cartilage cells initially become hypertrophic and then begin to die

✓ Hemopoetic cells (monocytes) arrive from liver or spleen and they finally become multinucleated osteoclasts

✓ Blood vessels are formed into the primary ossification centers

After these steps, the new blood vessels carry with them pericytes. Pericytes (or perivascular cells) are mesenchymal in origin and differentiate into osteoblasts on the surface of the calcified cartilage. This differentiation is the same as in intramembranous bone formation (they produce collagen, proteoglycans and matrix vesicles). Matrix vesicles are the initial calcification sites. Gradually they grow in size; they become bone nodules, woven bone and finally lamellar bone. So all what happens is the same as intramembranous bone formation. The only difference is that endochondreal osteogenesis occurs on a specule of calcified cartilage. The calcified cartilage plays <u>no</u> role in the development of bone in the outside. They are two separate entities. As osteogenesis goes on, bone marrow starts to develop in the medullary cavity. Epithelial growth disc is responsible for the growth of bone after birth. What happens in this disc is the same that happens in primary ossification centers. If we see a section of cartilage, we can distinguish certain layers:

✓ Resting layer (cells are replicating their DNA)

✓ Zone of proliferation

✓ Area of hypertrophy

✓ Area of calcification

✓ Area of calcified cartilaginous specules

✓ Area of chondroblasts

✓ Area of osteoclasts

✓ Areas of woven or lamellar bone

In each bone, two secondary ossification centers are found. What happens is the same as in primary ossification centers. The difference is in the morphology. As bone continues to grow, epiphysial disc becomes narrow and narrower. At the ages of 17-19 years, all cartilage is calcified and bone stops growing. Bone becomes trabecular and compact. Both of them are lamellar bone. It is difficult to distinguish them microscopically. A very small proportion of the initial cartilage is found in adult bone.

LAMELLAR BONE

Cartilage grows interstitially and appositionally on the bone surface.

Bone producing cells are found in:

✓ Periosteum (osteogenic layer)

✓ Endosteum

    -in the cortical area

    -in the trabecular area

✓ Osteons (old term: Haversian system)

Osteoblasts are found on these surfaces. If we do not find osteoblasts we see two kinds of cells:

✓ Osteoclasts

✓ Bone lining cells (like osteoblasts)

Live bone implies living cells on its surface. Organism gets rid of the necrotic bone by osteoclasts or macrophages.

Bone is a very well vascularized organ. Vascularization comes from the fibrous layer of periosteum, from the medullary cavity and from endosteum.

How does adult bone take its shape?

✓ Woven bone

✓ Lamellar bone

    -circumferential lamellae

    inner lamellae

    outer lamellae

    -concentric-osteonal (surrounding haversian canals)

✓ Interstitial bone

✓ Trabecular lamellae

Volksman canals carry blood vessels in the Haversian canals. Collagen and trabecular lamellae are parallel; they have the same orientation.

Osteoid is defined as the uncalcified matrix. Osteoblasts are always found close to blood vessels, because they function as agents helping the nutrition of bone.

Histology-Embryology of Osteons

Continuous apposition of bone is taking place inside the growing osteon. As more matrix is laid down and is calcified, cells are entraped inside the matrix. These cells are called osteocytes. Osteocytes reside in the lacunae. The difference between cartilaginous cells and bone cells inside the matrix, is that cartilaginous cells get their nutrients through diffusion while osteocytes through canaliculi. Canaliculi communicate with osteoblasts at the surface of bone with gap junctions. Since osteoblasts are close to blood vessels, canaliculi are believed to help nutrition.

As for the mature osteon, several lamellae and numerous osteocytes and canaliculi are observed. Outside the osteon we can see a line. This line is called cement line and joins two osteons as they start to form. There is also another kind of cement line, the rest or reverse line, which is a point where resorption has stopped.

The arteries that invade in the primary ossification center of the diaphesis are named nutrient or diaphesial arteries. The arteries that enter in the secondary ossification center in the epiphysis are named epiphysial arteries. Metaphysial arteries are the arteries in the metaphysis (neck of the bone). There are also numerous bone marrow arteries.

BONE AND BONE MARROW CELLS

The more embryonic a cell is the less it can do, but the more potential it has for doing many different things. The more primitive a cell is, the more lightly is stained in histologic sections. Euchromatin is representative of the DNA in the nucleus. The more euchromatin a cell has, the more potentiality that cell has. The presence of euchromatin indicates less differentiation. Heterochromatin indicates more differentiation. Differentiation has also reflection on cytoplasm. Well-differentiated cells have bigger cytoplasm and large Golgi apparatus, which secretes glycoproteins, proteoglycans and glycosoaminoglucans. They also have increased numbers of mitochondria (energy production sites) and increased amounts of rough endoplasmic reticulum.

The primitive cells of bone are mesenchymal cells, then they become osteoprogenitor cells and finally they become osteoblasts. Osteoprogenitor cells are the major dividing cells of bone. Osteoblasts under normal circumstances do not further divide.

We see bone formation in embryonic life. What happens in adult life or in other words, what we carry from embryonic life?

We mainly carry three categories of cells:

✓ Pericytes or perivascular cells. These cells are candidate for the mesenchymal cell.

✓ Stromal cells. They are found in bone marrow and they originate from connective tissue. They are a source of osteoblasts.

✓ Colony forming unit of bone (CFU_o) ($_o$ indicates osteogenesis). They are hemopoetic stem cells in bone marrow. They are considered to give rise to all bone marrow originating cells (erythrocytes, lymphocytes, monocytes, neutrophils, basophils, eosinophils, mast cells)

Osteocytes are formed from osteoblasts. They are encircled cells and they are found in their lacunae.

Osteoblasts are found in the surface. According to their secretory activity, they are subdivided into resting or active osteoblasts. Resting osteoblasts look like fibroblasts [2]. Osteoclasts are multinucleated cells (up to 50-100 nuclei). Howship's lacunae (resorption cavities) can be seen around them. They have many lysosomes.

BONE ABSORPTION

Osteoclasts produce collagenases, carbohydrases and proteinases to break down collagen, carbohydrates and proteins. At the same time, they produce acids, which lower the pH. The result is the breakdown of hydroxyapatite.

Then, under the guidance of parathyroid hormone which stimulates osteoclasts and encourages them to begin the process of absorption, osteoclasts uptake Ca^{++} and P^{+++} ions with endocytosis and they secrete them to the vascular system with exocytosis. Finally, we have resorption cavities in the bone (Howship's lacunae) and we get Ca^{++} and P^{+++} back to the blood circulation.

In the bone marrow, we see fat cells and blood vessels. We also see small blood vessels called sinusoids, which enter the bone.

ORIGIN AND DEVELOPMENT OF OSTEOBLASTS AND OSTEOCLASTS

Mesenchymal cells differentiate into osteoprogenitor cells, which then differentiate into osteoblasts.

Osteoblasts form a spheroid membrane of cells and secrete inside this sphere:

- collagen

- non-collagenous proteins

- glucosoaminoglycans

- matrix vesicles

Matrix vesicles are the initial calcifications loci. Hydroxyapatite crystals grow from the matrix vesicles into small spheroid formations, called bone nodules.

Bone nodules coalesce into seams of woven bone. Osteoblasts secrete oriented collagen now without matrix vesicles.

Hydroxyapatite now grows directly into, onto and between collagen fibrils initiating lamellar bone formation.

HORMONAL EFFECTS IN CA^{++} HOMEOSTASIS

Ninety nine percent of Ca^{++} is stored in bone. Only 1% is found in cells, serum and in extracellular fluids. Half of this 1% is bound in citrates, phosphates or other substances (ionized form). Ca^{++} is also important component of hydroxyapatite. The density of Ca^{++} in serum is 10% [3,4].

Calcium homeostasis is very important because it is essential for holding cells together, for muscle activity and nerve impulse.

When the density of Ca^{++} is lowered in plasma, the chief cells of parathyroid glands are stimulated and they secrete parathyroid hormone.

Three major hormones affect Ca^{++} homeostasis [5-10]:

✓ Parathyroid hormone

✓ Calcitonin

✓ Vitamin D

There are also some other factors, like growth hormone, whose role is more important for the formation of cartilage.

Features of Parathyroid Hormone

✓ It is produced in chief cells of parathyroid glands and is released into the blood stream

✓ It has effects on all bone cells

-osteoclasts: helps osteoclasts to begin bone absorption

-osteocytes: helps osteocytes to begin an "osteocytic osteolysis"

-osteoblasts: helps osteoblasts to become resorptive cells

✓ It has effects on tubule cells of the kidney [11]

-helps reabsorption of Ca^{++}

-helps absorption of phosphates

-helps hydroxylization of vitamin D_3

Features of Calcitonin

✓ It is produced by the clear cells of thyroid gland

✓ Turns off the cells on which parathormone has already acted (opposite effect of parathormone) [12,13]

✓   It does not increase bone deposition

✓   It has effects on osteoblasts and osteoclasts and keeps them down from resorpting the bone

✓   Dual feedback system:

-parathyroid hormone: raises Ca^{++} level in blood

-calcitonin: lowers Ca^{++} level in blood [14,15]

Characteristics of Vitamin D

Vitamin D is a group of fat-soluble prohormones, the two major forms of which are vitamin D_2 (or ergocalciferol) and vitamin D_3 (or cholecalciferol). We get vitamin D through food and sunlight. Its active form is dihydroxycalciferol (vit.D_3) [16-22].

Vitamin D_3 is like parathyroid hormone.

✓   It raises Ca^{++} level in the blood.

✓   Promotes absorption of calcium and phosphorus from food in the intestines, and reabsorption of calcium in the kidneys. As a steroid hormone, it acts on the nucleus of the cells. Parathormone helps Ca^{++} to get into the cell, while vitamin D_3 helps transport through the cell [23].

✓   It is necessary for bone growth and bone remodeling by osteoblasts and osteoclasts.

✓   It affects osteoblasts in tissue culture, causing them to form junctional complexes [24].

Characteristics of Other Hormones

Thyroxin: It increases metabolism of all cells. It has net effect on deposition of bone

Clucocorticosteroids: They decrease collagen synthesis and have negative effect on bone formation

Growth hormone: Its major effect is on the epiphyseal growth plate

Androgens - Estrogens: They have protective effect on bone. Lack of estrogens leads to osteoporosis

Prostaglandines: They play a role in bone resorption

REMODELING OF BONE

Modeling of bone is the process in which embryological bone changes its size and develops to adult bone.

It is characterized by:

✓   change in size

✓   change in position (drift)

✓   change in shape (for some bones)

In the modeling process, every bone surface (periosteum, cortical endosteum, trabecular endosteum and osteonal endosteum) is involved. Approximately 95% of these surfaces are involved in modeling.

Remodeling is the change of bone surface in some punctuated areas. The changes of remodeling occur in less than 20% of bone surfaces.

Remodeling is characterized by two functions:

✓   resorption of bone

✓   deposition of bone

In young ages: deposition > resorption

In medium age: deposition = resorption

In late part of life: resorption > deposition (osteoporosis)

Why do we have remodeling?

✓   to maintain calcium equilibrium

✓   to respond to stress

Depositional cells   =   osteoblasts

Resorption cells   =   osteoclasts

Resorption must take place in order the bone to maintain its normal structure. If resorption does not occur (eg inhibition with bisphosphonates), osteopetrosis might occur.

COUPLING PHENOMENON

Resorption usually precedes deposition of bone in the remodeling process. Initially osteoclasts develop, they resorb the bone, a Howship's lacuna is formed and osteoclasts disappear. Migration of intermediate stem cells then occurs, osteoblasts are formed and finally bone is produced.

Diagrammatically, coupling phenomenon has as follows:

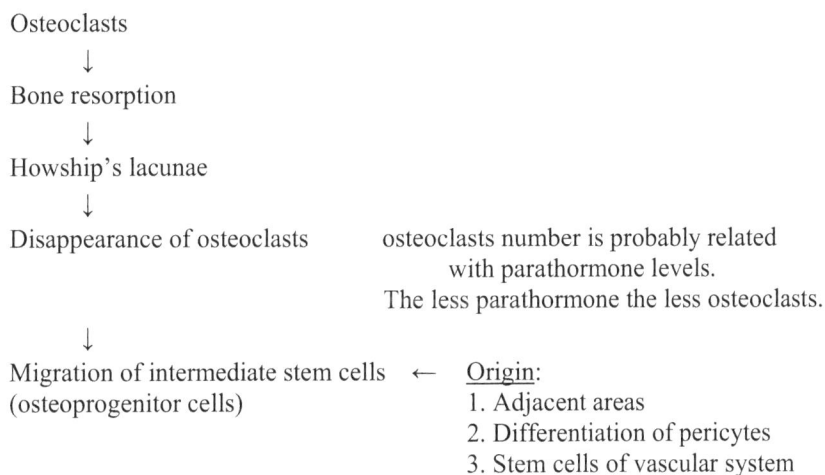

Osteoclasts
↓
Bone resorption
↓
Howship's lacunae
↓
Disappearance of osteoclasts   osteoclasts number is probably related
                                                        with parathormone levels.
                                        The less parathormone the less osteoclasts.

↓
Migration of intermediate stem cells   ←   Origin:
(osteoprogenitor cells)   1. Adjacent areas
                                                2. Differentiation of pericytes
                                                3. Stem cells of vascular system

Now let us look at individual sites of bone and see how remodeling takes place:

On the surface: A blood vessel grows close to the resorbed area and carries cells, which differentiate to osteoblasts that will produce new bone. Finally, we have an osteon canal with blood vessels inside and concentric lamellae around it and the cement line around the osteon (closing cone).

In areas with stress: When stress is applied to bone, resorption takes place. The trabecular bone patterns are also configured according to the direction of stress forces. In several cases, trabecular patterns are formed as gothic arches.

PHYSIOLOGY OF BONE

We will mainly focus on collagen formation, proteoglycans interactions and on process of calcification

Collagen

They are 10-12 different types of collagen. We will talk about 4 of them.

Type I: It is mainly found in the skin, bone, tendons, ligaments, dentin and cementum.

Type II: It is a thinner form and is mainly found in cartilage

Type III: It is mainly found in the connective and fetal tissue

Press IV: It is located in the basal lamina (portion of basement membrane)

The molecule of collagen consists of a triple helix. The differences of these four types are in the helixes (a and b helixes)

Procollagen is a final product of the endoplasmic reticulum of collagen-producing cells.

Osteoblasts and other cells produce collagen.

Schematically the production of collagen has as follows:

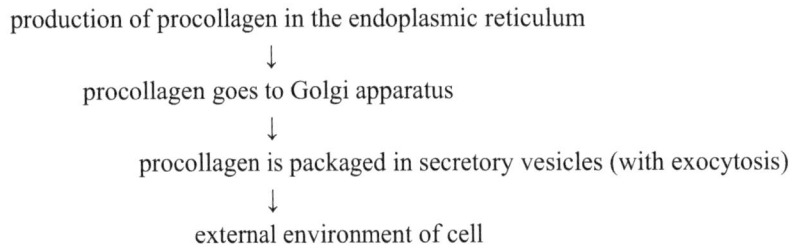

production of procollagen in the endoplasmic reticulum
↓
procollagen goes to Golgi apparatus
↓
procollagen is packaged in secretory vesicles (with exocytosis)
↓
external environment of cell

Procollagen has two peptide ends, which are cleaved off.

Why are these two peptide ends significant?

✓   they aloud the formation of triple helix
✓   they aloud the transportation outside the cell
✓   they aloud polymerization through cleaving off

During polymerization, we have reactions between different tropocollagen molecules. One result of polymerization is the formation of microfibrills. Microfibrills are accumulations of five collagen molecules side to side.

After that, we have formation of collagen fibers. The strength of collagen is the same as steel.

Proteoglycans Interactions

They are located among collagen fibers. Their molecule is very huge and has a core mainly consisting of proteins. Chondroitin and hyaluronic acid are found in attached form. There is also a link protein joining core proteins and hyaluronic acid. Calcium ions pass through proteoglycans.

One question is since we have type I collagen in many tissues why mineralization occurs only in bone, dentin and cementum? The answer is that in these tissues interactions with other factors may take place. An important factor is the presence of matrix vesicles in mineralized tissues. There are also enzymes, such as alkaline phosphatase, either in the matrix vesicles or in bone that initiate the mineralization process.

Process of Calcification

Calcium ions exhibit an affinity of attaching to the mineralized tissues. They enter into the bone through channels that line the bone surface. Ca^{++} can return to the extracellular fluid through lining cells of bone surface (resorption). Generally, they enter or exit according to bone needs. Parathyroid hormone increases the entry of Ca^{++} in blood.

Hydroxylapatite

Hydroxylapatite, also called hydroxyapatite, is a naturally occurring <u>mineral</u> form of calcium <u>apatite</u>. It is a crystal (3 dimensional structure). Its chemical type is: $Ca_{10}(PO_4)_6(OH)_2$. It grows with apposition of ions.

The very first nucleus of hydroxyapatite is formed:

✓ homogeneously or

✓ heterogeneously

Up to fifty percent of <u>bone</u> is made up of a modified form of the inorganic mineral hydroxyapatite. Carbonated-calcium deficient hydroxyapatite is the main mineral of which <u>dental enamel</u> and <u>dentin</u> are comprised.

PRIMARY AND SECONDARY CALCIFICATION

Primary calcification takes place in tissues that calcification of woven bone have never taken place before. It takes place in matrix vesicles. Secondary calcification is subsequent to the primary calcification. It occurs in a tissue where primary calcification has left a mass of calcified tissue. Primary calcification starts in the matrix vesicles of the embryonal bone (mesenchymal cells), the crystals continue to grow and they coalesce into woven bone. This procedure takes place whether bone formation is intramembranous or endochondreal. Wherever bone is formed, it is formed exactly with this way. Later on, the cells after a genetic signal stop to produce matrix vesicles and they begin to produce oriented collagen. Calcification now occurs on the collagen fibers from the initial crystal masses of the primary calcification. This kind of calcification is called secondary. Primary and secondary calcification is related to primary (woven) and secondary (lamellar) bone. Primary and secondary bones are the embryonic events that take place in the development of a tissue. Primary and secondary calcification is the events that take place through the mineralization of that tissue. In cartilage, we have primary calcification as we have in woven bone. Cartilaginous cells produce matrix vesicles, which are the initial sites of calcification. After that, we have formation of cartilaginous nodules, same as bone nodules. The tooth consists of three calcified tissues; enamel, dentin and cementum. Embryologically, ameloblasts are first formed and then they induce the formation of odontoblasts. Odontoblasts are the first calcification sites. Ameloblasts are then calcified (enamel waits for dentin to be calcified). Ameloblasts – odontoblasts are characterized as a reciprocal inductive system. After that, cementum is induced to be calcified. The matrix secreted by odontoblasts induces cementoblasts to form cementum, which is then subjected to calcification. Primary calcification occurs in mantle dentin. Secondary calcification occurs in circumpulpal dentin, enamel and cementum.

Generally, we have:

Primary calcification	Secondary calcification
- woven bone	- lamellar bone
- calcified cartilage	- circumpulpal dentin
- mantle dentin	- enamel
	- cementum

Mechanisms of Calcification

There is an active transform of calcium in the matrix vesicles. This is energized by a calcium-ATPase system. This ATPase system is an alkaline phosphatase. Alkaline phosphatase includes a broad spectrum of isoenzymes. One of those isoenzymes is ATPase. ATPase is located on cell membranes. ATPase helps for the development of hydroxylapatite.

There is also another isoenzyme, the phosphoesterase, which is also alkaline phosphatase. It is located in the matrix vesicles. It promotes the release of phosphate ions, useful for the development of hydroxyapatite.

Another isoenzyme is pyrophosphatase, which breaks down pyrophosphates. Pyrophosphates are inhibitory to the calcification mechanisms. Alkaline phosphatase is related both to primary and secondary calcification.

OSTEOCLASTIC-OSTEOBLASTIC PATHOLOGY AND METABOLIC BONE DISEASES

Osteoclastic pathology

Osteoclasts are involved in many diseases. We will refer to three of them. Osteoclasts are multinucleated giant cells. Other multinucleated cells in bone marrow are the megakaryocytes that make the platelets. The origin of the osteoclast is not well known. Some believe that it originates from a circulating histiocyte. It starts as a mononuclear cell and then fusing with others it becomes multinucleated cell. These cells show no mitotic activity. Their principal function is to absorb bone. They dissolve bone with acid phosphatases, as well as with collagenases. Three main diseases in which osteoclast function is abnormal are the following:

Osteopetrosis

In normal adults, osteoclasts are working in the metaphysis. Osteopetrosis is a systemic disease in which, due to genetic factors, osteoclasts are not working. Osteoclasts fail to destroy bone as well as calcified cartilage. Osteoclasts are present in osteopetrosis. The thing that is missing is osseous lacunae. Osteopetrosis can range from mild to severe. The rate of mortality depends on the severity of the disease. Bone in osteopetrosis appears radioopaque.

Due to narrowing of the bone marrow cavity the patient is subjected to anemias, infections etc. Therapeutically irradiations of the whole body or bone marrow transplantation are the treatments of choice.

Hyperparathyroidism

The function of parathormone is to keep calcium levels elevated. Calcium is important for nerves and muscles. Most of the calcium (99%) is stored in the bones. One of the main symptoms of elevated calcium is depression of neuromuscular electrical function. Diagnosis of hyperparathyroidism is established in the laboratory (high Ca^{++} and alkaline phosphatase levels, low P^{+++} levels).

Elevated calcium levels lead to deposition of stones in various organs (e.g. kidney). The most dramatic changes of hyperparathyroidism occur in bones (tumors). Lamina dura of teeth disappears. Giant cell tumors also occur in the oral cavity.

Cortical resorption and increased fibroblastic activity occurs in bone tumors of hyperparathyroidism. Bone tumors of hyperparathyroidism are also called brown tumors. Brown tumors occur in the metaphysis or diaphesis of bones. They are full of hyperactive osteoclasts.

Giant cell tumors also occur. They are found in the metaphysis of bones.

Paget's Disease

Typically is found in Europeans (especially Germans). It was thought that this disease was due to osteoblastic hypoactivity, but this proved to be wrong.

Today it is believed that Paget's disease is a slow viral infection that causes osteoclastic proliferation. Osteoclastic proliferation causes bone destruction. The classic model is that osteoclasts create a mosaic pattern. The responsible virus probably belongs to the paramyxoviruses group, including the measles virus.

The classical symptoms of the disease are

- ✓ enlargement of head
- ✓ deafness
- ✓ blindness

Microscopically the picture is similar to hyperparathyroidism. Blood chemistry is normal.

There is also a predisposition of Paget's disease lesions to development of sarcoma. Ten percent of the patients develop osteogenic sarcoma.

Osteoblastic Pathology

Diseases affecting the function of osteoblasts are:

Osteogenesis Imperfecta

Osteogenesis imperfecta (sometimes known as Brittle bone disease or Lobstein syndrome) is a genetic bone disorder. As a genetic disorder, it has an autosomal dominant defect. Most people with Osteogenesis imperfecta receive it from a parent but it can be an individual mutation. It is usually characterized by deficiency of Type-I collagen. Osteoblasts do not have the capacity to make lamellar bone. They stay in embryonal condition. Therefore, there is a defect in collagen (type I) production.

There are two major forms of osteogenesis imperfecta:

✓ pure genetic (all genes affected)
✓ some genes are affected, some not

Usually in the age of 3 all woven bone is replaced by lamellar bone. That does not happen in this disease.

Blood chemistry is normal.

The symptoms depend on the ratio of lamellar/woven bone.

Osteoporosis

Osteoporosis is a pathologic situation caused by chronic protein deficiency of bone. It affects more than 20 million individuals in the United States. Over than 150,000 suffer from femoral fractures and 1/6 of them die due to the consequences of immobilization.

Risk factors of osteoporosis:

➢ well established factors (increased risk)
  - Sex (female)
  - Caucasians, Asian race, not Blacks
  - Small skeleton
  - Premenopausal oophorectomy
  - Glucocorticoid consumption
  - Immobility
  - Hypoestrogenemia
➢ Factors with moderate evidence (increased risk)
  - Positive family
  - Low calcium intake
  - Alcoholism
  - Smoking
  - Caffeine (little evidence)
  - Heparin treatment

> Factors decreasing the risk

- Blacks

- Obesity

- Women in menopause receiving estrogen therapy

- Good life style factors (diet, exercise)

Types of osteoporosis:

	Juvenille
Primary	Idiopathic
	Involutional

	Endocrine diseases
	Gastrointestinal diseases
Secondary	Bone marrow diseases
	Connective tissue diseases
	Miscellaneous causes

Diagnosis of osteoporosis:

The simple radiographs are not useful since they do not reveal any bone changes unless we have 30% or more bone loss.

Bone density measurements are widely used. They include:

✓ Single photon absorptiometry (not very sensitive)

✓ Dual photon absorptiometry

✓ CT and MRI tomography (very sensitive)

Bone fractures usually occur. People may loose five inches of their original height. Osteoporosis is a condition that cannot be reversed. There is normal blood chemistry.

Histopathology of osteoporosis:

One third of the patients show low turnover or inactive osteopenia. This means that the rate of remodeling is slow. Few osteoblasts, few osteoclasts and not much osteoid are observed.

Another one third of the osteoporotic patients show accelerated rate of bone formation. High turnover or active osteopenia is observed in these cases. Numerous osteoblasts, osteoclasts and osteoid are seen.

In the last one third of patients, the features are ranging.

Other organ systems that contribute to the development of osteoporosis are:

✓ Parathyroid hormone levels

✓ Calcium absorption (in the gut)

✓ Kidney (production of hydroxy-vitamin D)

✓ Kidney (how much calcium goes out to urine)

✓ Sex steroids

Therapeutic agents of osteoporosis:

➢ Factors increasing bone formation

  - NaF

  - Exercise

  - Testosterone

  - Vitamin D_2

  - Oral -PO_4

➢ Agents decreasing bone resorption

  - Estrogens

  - Anabolic steroids

  - Testosterone

  - Calcitonin

  - Vitamin D_2

  - Oral -PO_4

  - Bisphosphonates

  - Oral calcium

Osteomalacia

Osteomalacia is a decrease in mineralized bone mass, due to the inability to mineralize the osteoid. What we see is increased amounts of osteoid.

In most cases of osteomalacia, there is an underlying renal or gastrointestinal disease. Usually there is calcium or vitamin D deficiency, either from intestine malabsorption or from not enough milk intake or insufficient exposure to sunlight. In osteomalacia, there is an increase of osteoid, which is produced by osteoblasts. Osteomalacia occurring in childhood is named rickets.

In rickets, we have swellings in joints. The presence of cartilage and polysaccharides that absorb water, in the metaphysis, explains the swellings in joints.

Osteomalacia is a condition that most physicians say, "we need a bone biopsy".

The histological types of osteomalacia are:

✓ Type I: There is increase of osteoid, increased numbers of osteoblasts and osteoclasts. It is found in vitamin D deficiency, malabsorption syndromes, pathologic conditions with liver and kidney metabolism, rickets and Paget's disease.

✓ Type II: There is increased presence of osteoid, increased numbers of osteoblasts, no increase of osteoblasts, no bone marrow fibrosis.

✓ Type III: Increased amount of osteoid and few osteoblasts are present in this type of osteomalacia. It is mainly found in bone diseases related to kidney problems (renal osteodystrophy) and in malnutritional conditions.

Treatment of choice is the administration of vitamin D, immobilization (in case of fractures), prevention of infections and suggestions for exposure to sunlight.

Scurvy

Scurvy is a disease resulting from a deficiency of vitamin C, which is required for the synthesis of collagen in humans. Scurvy does not occur in most animals because they can synthesize their own vitamin C, but humans, other primates and a few other species lack an enzyme necessary for such synthesis and must obtain vitamin C through their diet. Scurvy leads to the formation of macular lesions on the skin, edematous gingiva, and bleeding from the mucous membranes. The macular lesions are most abundant on the thighs and legs, and most patients look pale, depressed, and are partially immobilized. In advanced scurvy, there are open, suppurating oral ulcers and loss of <u>teeth</u>.

In scurvy osteoblasts and collagen formation are mainly affected.

Microscopically, tiny trabecullae and osteoblast proliferation without osteoid formation are observed.

Osteogenic Sarcoma

It is probably the most frequent primary malignant tumor of bones. It occurs in young ages. It initially presents as a painless mass.

Microscopically is characterized by presence of:

- ✓ malignant osteoblasts
- ✓ osteoid
- ✓ anaplasia
- ✓ woven bone

Chemotherapy is the treatment of choice for osteogenic sarcoma.

FRACTURES AND FRACTURE REPAIR

In fractures, the beginning of healing occurs at the osteogenic layer of the periosteum. A fracture callus develops around bone, which is in fracture healing process. In fracture callus, there is a proliferation of cells, then formation of cartilage and finally formation of woven bone. There is external and internal fracture callus. There is also periosteal and endosteal bone formation.

Phases of fracture healing:

➤ Inflammatory
Hematoma formation
Osteocyte death
Vasodilation
Edema
Inflammatory cells

Disruption of blood supply

➤ Reparative
Bone necrosis
Ingrowth of vasoformative elements
Cellular proliferation
Pain and swelling
Vascular dilatation

➤ Bone remodeling
Vessel proliferation
Mesenchymal cell proliferation
Change of acid pH to alkaline
Collagen production
(initially type II, then type I)

The way that fractures heal with callus is similar with the way that occurs in endochondreal bone formation. It resembles the epiphyseal plate (histologically and biochemically).

Biochemical changes occurring in epiphyseal plate:

✓ Glycogen accumulation (when calcification occurs, glycogen disappears)

✓ Increase in total lipids (calcium phospholipids)

✓ Change from neutral to acid proteoglycans

✓ Increased levels of alkaline phosphatase

✓ Extracellular vesicles

Components of callus:

✓ Proteoglycans (high in the first two weeks, during the inflammatory phase)

✓ Collagen (initially all types, finally only type I)

✓ Minerals (hydroxyapatite, in bone formation phase)

Factors affecting fracture healing:

- **Age:** Young patients heal rapidly and have a remarkable ability to remodel and correct angulation's deformities. These abilities decrease once skeletal maturity is reached.

- **Nutrition:** A substantial amount of energy is needed for fracture healing to occur. Calcium promotes fracture healing. Excessive amounts of phosphate inhibit bone formation. Small amounts of fluoride increase bone formation while large amounts decrease bone formation. Decreased oxygen capacity delays bone formation. Generally, the role of nutrition on fracture healing is limited.

- **Systemic Diseases:** Diseases like osteoporosis, diabetes, and those causing an immunocompromised state will likely delay healing. Marfan's and Ehlers-Danlos syndromes cause abnormal musculoskeletal healing.

- **Hormones:** Cortisone, inhibits protein synthesis and affects calcium absorption in the gut, calcitonin inhibits bone resorption. It is considered to have a positive effect but in reality is a transitional factor. Growth hormone enhances bone formation but it has a very limited role in terms of clinical significance. Thyroxine plays an insignificant clinical role.

- **Type of bone:** Cancellous bone fractures are usually more stable, involve greater surface areas, and have a better blood supply than do cortical bone fractures. Cancellous bone heals faster than cortical bone.

- **Degree of Trauma:** The more extensive the injury to bone and surrounding soft tissue, the poorer the outcome.

- **Vascular Injury:** Inadequate blood supply impairs healing. Especially vulnerable areas are the femoral head, talus, and scaphoid bones.

- **Degree of Immobilization:** The fracture site must be immobilized for vascular ingrowth and bone healing to occur. Repeated disruptions of repair tissue, especially to areas with marginal blood supply or heavy soft tissue damage, will impair healing.

- **Intraarticular Fractures:** These fractures communicate with synovial fluid, which contains collagenases that retard bone healing.

- **Separation of Bone Ends:** Normal apposition of fracture fragments is needed for union to occur. Inadequate reduction, excessive traction, or interposition of soft tissue will prevent healing.

- **Infection:** Infections cause necrosis and edema, takes energy away from the healing process, and may increase the mobility of the fracture site.

Nutritional factors affecting fracture healing:

✓   Calcium (promotes fracture healing)

✓   Phosphate (excessive amounts of phosphate inhibit bone formation)

✓   Fluoride (small amounts increase bone formation while large amounts decrease bone formation)

Decreased oxygen capacity delays bone formation.

Bone Growth Factors

These factors can either induce or enhance bone formation

✓   Skeletal derived growth factor

✓   Transforming growth factor – B

✓   Fibroblast growth factor

✓   Platelet derived growth factor

✓   Bone morphogenetic protein

✓   Osteocyte induced factor

What growth factors do? They make induction.

Induction is the sum of processes that direct the differentiation of adjacent cells to restore function or regenerate structures. In other words, growth factors induce cells to become bone forming cells. More than one growth factors and sometimes some modulators are needed for this process.

BONE AND THE IMMUNE SYSTEM

There is a local as well as a systemic regulation of bone metabolism.

Growth factors are considered local factors and they have been shown to play an important role to bone metabolism.

Functions of growth factors:

✓   Stimulate cell proliferation

✓   Maintain cell viability

✓   Promote differentiation and development

✓   Help chemotaxis

✓   Activate inflammatory cells

✓   Play a role in tissue repair

✓   Play a role in disease states

What local factors do for bone?

✓   Stimulate or inhibit preosteoclasts and preosteoblasts

✓   Play a key role in coupling phenomenon

✓   <u>Mediate the effects of systemic hormones</u> (parathyroid hormone, hydroxyl vitamin D)

✓   Responsible for localized bone changes

The exact cellular source of many of these growth factors is not very well known.

There are two general subdivisions of growth factors; cytokines and prostaglandines.

Cytokines

They are believed to originate from activated lymphocytes.

Cytokines that have significant influence on osteoblasts or osteoclasts are:

- ✓ interferon γ
- ✓ transforming factor - β
- ✓ interkeukin 1
- ✓ tumor necrosis factor

Cytokines act on proliferation and differentiation of osteoclasts. Their action on bone is very complicated. Experimental observations on growth factors effects on bone have been performed in nude mice, which are insufficient of T lymphocytes. One of the older factors is the osteoclast-activating factor (OAF). It is released from human peripheral leukocytes. It activates osteoclasts and increases bone resorption.

Synthesis sites of growth factors:

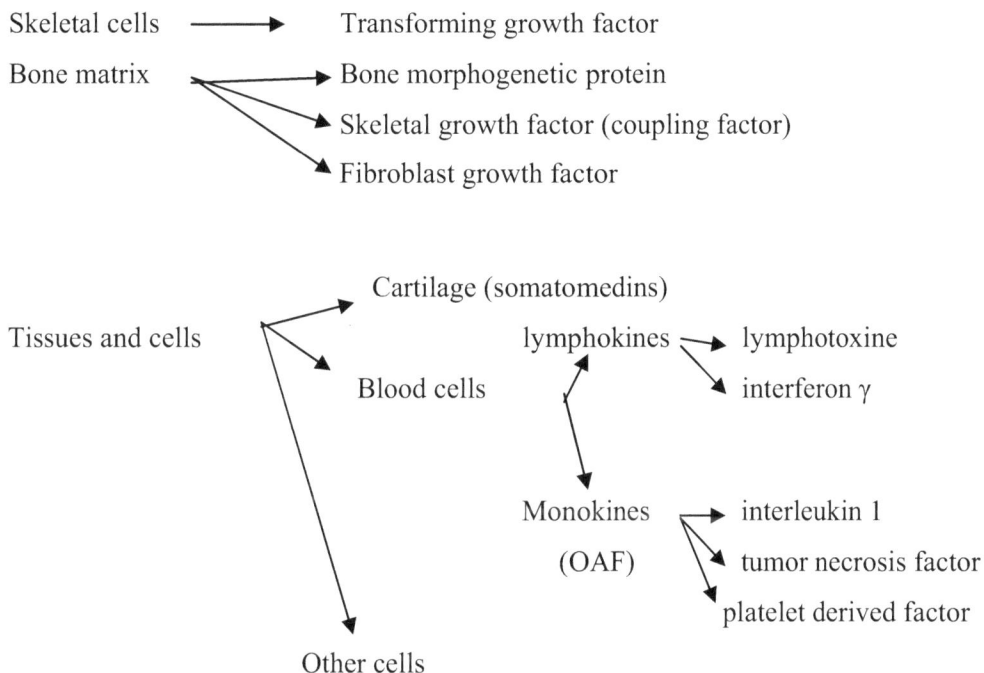

Skeletal cells ⟶ Transforming growth factor

Bone matrix → Bone morphogenetic protein
→ Skeletal growth factor (coupling factor)
→ Fibroblast growth factor

Tissues and cells → Cartilage (somatomedins)
→ Blood cells

lymphokines → lymphotoxine
→ interferon γ

Monokines
(OAF)

→ interleukin 1
→ tumor necrosis factor
→ platelet derived factor

Other cells

Functions of Interleukin 1

- ✓ stimulates bone cells
- ✓ causes bone resorption
- ✓ together with tumor necrosis factor causes breakdown and inhibit proteoglycan synthesis

Functions of tumor necrosis factor - α

- ✓ produced by activated macrophages
- ✓ cytostatic, cytolytic, antiviral effect
- ✓ stimulates bone resorption

Functions of transforming growth factor – β

- ✓ multifunctional regulator of bone
- ✓ influences extracellular matrix production

✓ plays significant role in interactions of epithelia and mesenchyme

✓ stimulates DNA synthesis and cell replication

✓ stimulates collagen synthesis

✓ parathyroid hormone releases transforming growth factor – β from bone. This is associated with coupling phenomenon.

Prostaglandines

Prostaglandines are unsaturated fatty acids. All mammalian cells can synthesize prostaglandins. Cells of the osteoblast lineage produce prostaglandins 1 and 2. Prostaglandins are also produced in bone and respond to inflammation, injuries, fractures etc.

Prostaglandins 1 and 2 stimulate bone resorption. We also know that administration of prostaglandins together with indomethacin inhibits fetal bone formation. Infusion of prostaglandin 1 induces striking periosteal new bone formation. High prostaglandin concentrations inhibit osteoblast collagen synthesis.

BONE ENHANCING FACTORS

Environmental factors are:

✓ nutrition (calcium intake is very important factor)

✓ drugs (estrogen treatment helps)

Components causing age related bone loss are:

✓ gonadal hormone loss: 25%/year bone loss

✓ senescence: 4%/year bone loss

✓ calcium deficiency: 1.5%/year bone loss

✓ other   variable

BONE AND IMPLANTS

Two basic problems related to implants are:

✓ what happens to the implant as it comes out to the oral mucosa

✓ what happens to implant in relation to the bone

We are going to be talking about the second, about the interface of implant to the bone, although these two problems are interrelated.

Two are the important questions for the implant; (a) can we put stable implants for a long time and (b) what are the biological factors in the implant – tissue interface?

When we deal with these questions, we have to deal with the whole process of osseointergration.

Numerous investigations regarding the interactions of implant – tissue interface have been performed [25].

Some of their most significant conclusions are the following:

✓ No osseointergration occurs with metallic implants

✓ A fibrous tissue layer is always present on metals

✓ True osseointergration occurs only in hydroxyapatite-coated implant

✓ Osteoblasts and bone matrix are only seen at the hydroxyapatite implant interface

✓ A non-ceramic (porous) hydroxyapatite coating on a solid core may be the most acceptable implant for clinical use

However, the research for ceramic hydroxyapatite is still ongoing.

REFERENCES

[1]   Donoghue PC, Sansom IJ. Origin and early evolution of vertebrate skeletonization. Microsc Res Tech 2002; 59: 352–72.

[2]   Caetano-Lopes J, Canhão H, Fonseca JE. Osteoblasts and bone formation. Acta Reumatológica Portuguesa 2007; 32: 103-10.

[3]   Brown EM. Physiology of Calcium Homeostasis. In: The Parathyroids, 2nd ed, Bilezikian JP, Marcus R, Levine A, Eds. New York, Raven Press, Chp 10, pp. 167-82, 2001.

[4]   Brown EM, Hebert SC. Calcium-receptor-regulated parathyroid and renal function. Bone 1997; 20:303-9.

[5]   Brown EM, Segre GV, Goldring SR. Serpentine receptors for parathyroid hormone, calcitonin and extracellular calcium ions. Baillieres Clin Endocrinol Metab 1996;10:123-61.

[6]   Deftos LJ. There's something fishy and perhaps fowl about the mammalian calcitonin receptor and its ligand. Endocrinology 1997; 138: 519-20.

[7]   Deftos, LJ. Clinical Essentials of Calcium and Skeletal Metabolism, Professional Communication Inc, 1st ed, 1998, pp. 1-208.

[8]   Deftos, LJ: Immunoassays for PTH and PTHrP In: The Parathyroids, 2nd ed, Bilezikian JP, Marcus R, Levine A, Eds, New York, Raven Press, Chp 9, pp.143-65, 2001.

[9]   Deftos, LJ. Hypercalcemia in malignant and inflammatory diseases. Endocrinol Metab Clin N Am 2002; 31:1-18.

[10]   Yanagawa N, Lee DBN: Renal Handling of Calcium and Phosphorus. In: Disorders of Bone and Mineral Metabolism, Coe FL, Favus MJ, Eds, 1992, Chapter 1, pp 3-40.

[11]   Berger UV, Peng JB, Hedier MA. The membrane transporter families in mammals. In: The Kidney, 3rd ed, Seldin DW, Giebisch G, Eds, Philadelphia, WB Saunders Co, Chp. 4, pp 107-38, 2000.

[12]   Deftos LJ and Gagel R. Calcitonin and Medullary Thyroid Carcinoma In: Cecil Textbook of Medicine, 21st ed, Philadelphia, WB Saunders Co, JB Wyngarden JB, Bennett JC, Chp 265, pp.1406-9, 2000.

[13]   Deftos LJ, Weisman MH, Williams GW, *et al.* Influence of age and sex on plasma calcitonin human beings. N Engl J Med 1980; 302:1351-3.

[14]   McLatchie LM, Fraser NJ, Main MJ, *et al.* RAMPs regulate the transport and ligand specificity of the calcitonin-receptor-like receptor. Nature 1998; 393: 333-9.

[15]   Muff R, Born W, Fischer JA. Calcitonin, calcitonin gene-related peptide, adrenomedullin and amylin: homologous peptides, separate receptors and overlapping biological actions. Eur J Endocrinol 1995; 133:17-20.

[16]   Bell NH. Renal and nonrenal 25-hydroxyvitamin D-1a-hydroxylases and their clinical significance. J Bone Miner Res 1998; 13:350-3.

[17]   Bruder JM, Guise TA, Mundy GR. Mineral Metabolism. In: Endocrinology & Metabolism, Fourth Edition, Felig P, Frohman LA, Eds, 2001, Chp 22, pp. 1079-1159.

[18]   Drezner, MK. Phosphorus Homeostasis and Related Disorders. In: Principles of Bone Biology, 2nd ed, JP Bilezikian JP , LG Raisz LG, Rodan GA, Eds, New York, Academic Press, Chp 22, pp 321-38, 2002.

[19]   Favus MJ: Intestinal Absorption of Calcium, Magnesium, and Phosphorus. In: Disorder of Bone and Mineral Metabolism, New York, Raven Press Coe FL, Favus MJ, Eds, Chp 3, pp 57-82, 1992.

[20]   Haussler MR, Whitfield GK, Haussler CA, et al. The nuclear vitamin D receptor: biological and molecular regulatory properties revealed. J Bone Miner Res 1998; 13: 325-49.

[21]   Holick, MF. Photobiology and Noncalcemic Actions of Vitamin D. In: Principles of Bone Biology, 2nd ed, New York, Academic Press, Bilezikian JP, Raisz LG, Rodan GA, Eds, Chp33, pp 587-602, 2002.

[22]   Knecht TP, Behling CA, Burton DW et al. The humoral hypercalcemia of benignancy. A newly appreciated syndrome. Am J Clin Pathol 1996; 105:487-92.

[23]   Nemere I, Farach-Carson MC. Membrane receptors for steroid hormones: a case for specific cell surface binding sites for vitamin D metabolites and estrogens. Biochem Biophys Res Commun 1998; 248:443-49.

[24]   Lacey DL, Timms E, Tan HL, et al. Osteoprotegerin ligand is a cytokine that regulates osteoclast differentiation and activation. Cell 1998; 93:165-76.

[25]   Ruano R, Jaeger RG, Jaeger MMM. Effect of a ceramic and a non-ceramic hydroxyapatite on cell growth and procollagen synthesis of cultured human gingival fibroblasts. J Periodontol 2000; 71: 540-5.

CHAPTER 3

Functions of Oral Mucosa

Anastasios K. Markopoulos

Aristotle University of Thessaloniki

Abstract: Oral mucosa shows specializations, which allow it to fulfill several roles. It protects mechanically against both compressive and shearing forces. It provides a barrier to micro-organisms, toxins and various antigens. It has a role in immunological defense, both humoral and cell-mediated. Minor glands within the oral mucosa provide lubrication and buffering as well as secretion of some antibodies. The mucosa is richly innervated, providing input for touch, proprioception, pain and taste. All these functions of oral mucosa are the main constituents of this chapter.

PROTECTIVE FUNCTION

The protective function of oral mucosa has two parts: the mechanical protection of the underlying tissues and the prevention of passage of microorganisms, toxic derivatives or other harmful substances.

The protective function is carried out with non-specific and specific resistance.

Non-specific resistance includes natural and cellular barriers.

In the natural barriers are included:

- the integrity of stratified squamous cell oral epithelium

- the antimicrobial factors that are present in the saliva

- the physiologic microbial flora that rivals the pathogenic micro-organisms

The phenomenon of inflammation is considered a cellular barrier.

Specific reaction is mainly carried out by the immune reaction, which is subdivided into cellular and humoral type.

RESISTANCE TO DISEASE

Two types of reactions contribute to the development of resistance against the disease, endogenous and adapted.

ENDOGENOUS = NON SPECIFIC

- General resistance against a wide spectrum of micro-organisms

- Direct reaction

- It develops in the place of appearance of the disease

Mechanisms: entire cellular membranes, phagocytes, antimicrobial substances inflammation

ADAPTED = SPECIFIC

- Specific reaction in the micro-organisms

- Slower in relation with the endogenous reaction

- It is acquired as long as the organism is exposed to the micro-organism

- Mechanisms: T lymphocytes, antibodies

- It protects from the pathogenic micro-organisms

- Isolation of cells and tissues that have suffered damage, infections or necrosis

- Identification of "self" from the foreign

Non Specific Resistance

✓ Natural barriers

✓ Cellular barriers

CELLULAR BARRIERS: INFLAMMATION

Functions of Inflammation:

- It deters the dissemination of micro-organisms in other tissues

- It removes the dead cells and the micro-organisms

- It prepares the tissues for repair

Signs and Symptoms of Inflammation:

- redness

- increase of temperature

- swelling

- pain

Main Chemical Substances of Inflammation

Histamine

- It is secreted by basophils and mast cells

- It causes vasodilation and increased vascular permeability

Quinines (proteins, eg bradykinin)

- It causes vasodilation and increased vascular permeability

- It causes chemotaxis (attraction of leukocytes in the region)

- Stimulate the pain receptors

Prostaglandines

- They sensitize the vessels for the action of other substances of inflamation

- They sensitize the pain receptors

Complement It promotes the inflammation

Cytokines

- Proteins that are produced by leukocytes or other cells

- Most of them promote the inflammation

Mechanisms of Inflammation

Vascular changes: vasodilation and increased vascular permeability that it results in:

- Hyperemia (increased blood flow in the region) and exit of plasma in the tissues

- Increase of temperature, increase of cellular metabolism

- Increase of oxygen and nutritious substances supply in the offended tissues and in the

- inflammatory cells

- Excretion of proteins that cause thrombosis
- Deters further dissemination of infection

Activation of phagocytes

- leukocytosis mainly neutrophils
- chemotaxis
- Adherence of phagocytes on the vascular wall
- Diapedesis (exit of phagocytes from the vessel)
- Phagocytosis of micro-organisms
- Pus formation usually in more serious infections

Neutrophils respond more fast (within a few hours)

- They are related with acute local inflammation

Monocytes respond slower (8-12 hours)

- They reach in the point of inflamation and are transformed in macrophages with numerous lysosomes
- They are related with chronic inflammation

Mechanisms of phagocytosis

Stages:

- ✓ Adherence of cell on the micro-organism

    -Recognition of micro-organism as "foreigner"

    -Phagocytosis is more difficult in micro-organisms with capsule

    -Opsonization Promotion of phagocytosis due to the presence of supplement and antibodies
- ✓ Formation of pseudopods and confinement of micro-organism in vesicles
- ✓ Lysosomal action on vesicles
- ✓ Digestion of micro-organism
- ✓ Exocytosis of undigested material

Cellular Barriers: Natural Killer Cells

- -Big granular lymphocytes
- -Responsible for the immune surveillance They react in the presence of non normal antigens
- -They destroy the neoplastic cells and cells infected from viruses
- -They release perforines

Perforines

- destroy the cellular membranes
- destroy the cell nuclei
- intensify the action of other substances

Antimicrobial Proteins: Compement

Group of approximately 20 proteins of serum circulating in inactive form [1].

Two ways of activation:

- Classic way
- It is related with the immune system

- Activation is result of interaction of antigen-antibody and certain basic proteins of
- complement
- Alternative way Interactions of proteins of complement with microbial wall
- polysaccharides

Both ways cause reactions that they result in:

- Increase of the non specific and specific resistance and intensification of inflammation and

Opsonization

- Destruction of bacterial cells

Antimicrobial Proteins: INTERFERONS

- Proteins that are secreted by cells infected by viruses

Interferons a and b, promote the synthesis of special proteins in adjacent non infected cells which inhibits proteinic synthesis in ribosomes and prevents viral replication

Interferon γ stimulates macrophages and natural killer cells

They can be produced in the laboratory and be used for therapeutic applications

Antimicrobial Proteins

Lysozyme: It is found in saliva and tears. It easily destroys microorganisms without capsule.

Specific Resistance

It is directed in certain antigens

It is systematic

It differentiates "same" from the "foreign" antigen

It has memory

Types

Humoral = immunity related with antibodies

B lymphocytes → plasma cells

Cellular = cellular type immunity

T lymphocytes

Antigens

Structures that activate the immune system

- Immunogenicity The property of a substance making it capable of inducing a detectable
- immune response
- Immunoreactivity the reaction with antibody, if this exists

Antigenic determinants = epitopes

- Regions of antigens that are recognized by the T lymphocytes and the antibodies
- Usually proteinic in nature

Complete antigens: They are also characterized by immunogenicity and by the presence of antigenic determinants

- Big molecules with > 1 antigenic determinants

-     Proteins, nucleic acids, lipids, polysaccharides

Haptens: they have antigenic determinants but are not immunogenic. However, they can react with an antibody of appropriate specificity.

-     Small molecules

-     They may be combined with other molecules in order to become complete antigens e.g. penicillin

Autoantigens= self antigens proteins of the major histocompatibility complex (MHC)

-     They are glycoproteins that are found in the cells of organism

-     Two types:

Class I they are found in every cell

Class II they are found in the cells that are involved in the immune reactions

TERMINOLOGY

Agglutination An antigen-antibody reaction in which a solid antigen forms a lattice with a soluble antibody

Precipitation A reaction between a soluble antigen and a soluble antibody in which a complex lattice of interlocking aggregates forms

Neutralization The antibody or antibody in complement covers active regions of antigen.

Cells of the Immune System

Lymphocytes

They become immunocompetent cells in the primary lymphatic organs (bone marrow and thymus) where they also learn to present immunotolerance. They migrate to the secondary lymphatic bodies in order to react with the exogenic antigens

Types:

-     B cells = B lymphocytes

-     T cells = T lymphocytes

-     Antigen presenting cells

B lymphocytes

-     They become immunocompetent cells in the bone marrow

-     After antigenic irritation they are differentiated into plasma cells and produce antibodies

T lymphocytes

-     They become immunocompetent cells in the thymus gland

-     They participate in the cellular immunity

Antigen Presenting Cells

Types:

-     Dendritic cells

-     Langerhans cells

-     Macrophages

-     Activated B lymphocytes

-     They present antigens to T lymphocytes

Humoral Immunity

Humoral immunity is carried out from B lymphocytes

Initial reaction The antigen is connected with the B lymphocyte

B lymphocyte is divided in daughter cells that secrete the antibodies or become mnemonic cells

Secondary reaction it is faster due to the presence of mnemonic cells

Antibodies

Immunoglobulins (Igs) = g-globulin

General structure:

-   They consist of four polypeptide chains that are linked with disulphide bonds
-   Each chain has a constant and variable region

Variable region

-   It determines the specificity of antibody
-   It contains the sites of antigen adherence

Constant region

-   It contains regions with heavy chains and regions with heavy and light chains
-   The regions with heavy chains determine the class of antibody

Classes of Antibodies

IgG

-   The most abundant antibody in plasma
-   It protects from bacteria, viruses, toxins
-   It activates the complement
-   It passes through placenta to protect fetus

IgM

-   It acts as antigenic receptor in the membrane of B of lymphocytes
-   It causes agglutination
-   It activates the supplement

IgA

-   It is mainly found in various secretions (saliva, sweat, milk, mucous secretions)
-   It deters the bacterial adherence on the epithelial cells

IgD

-   It acts as antigenic receptor

IgE

-   It is found in the skin, mucous membranes
-   It is connected with mast cells and basophiles
-   It is increased in the allergic reactions and in parasitic infections

Mechanisms of action of antibodies

They increase phagocytosis causing:

- neutralization

- agglutination

- precipitation

They activate the supplement, which:

- increases the inflammation

- destroys the cellular membranes

- increases phagocytosis

Cellular Immunity

Participation of T cells

Types of T Cells

- Cytotoxic T cells (T_C)

- Helper T cells (T_H)

- Suppressor T cells (T_S)

- T cells of delayed hypersensitivity (T_{DH})

Cytotoxic T Cells (T_C)

They destroy cells that are infected by some antigen

They destroy neoplastic cells

How their action is performed:

- releasing cytokines

- producing lymphotoxins (they destroy bacterial DNA)

- releasing tumor necrosis factor (TNF; It destroys the bacterial cell)

- with γ interferons (stimulate macrophages)

Helper T Cells (T_H)

They contribute to the production: of B lymphocytes and cytotoxic T cells

Other Types of T Cells

Suppressor T cells (T_S) they limit the activity of T and B cells after the confrontation of infection

T cells of Delayed Hypersensitivity (T_{DH})

- They participate in reactions of delayed hypersensitivity secreting interferons and other cytokines

- They promote non specific phagocytosis through macrophages

Activation of T Cells

1st stage binding with the antigen

The antigenic receptor of T cell binds with the antigen and his major histocombatibility complex (MHC) protein 2nd stage Simultaneous stimulation

The complex produced in the 1st stage causes production and activation of various types of T cells

Cytokines

- They are released from T cells and macrophages

MOLECULAR AND CELLULAR BASE OF IMMUNOPROTECTION THAT IS PROVIDED BY ORAL CAVITY

Oral cavity is a region susceptible to colonization and infiltration by microorganisms. The quantity of sIgA exceeds the total amounts of circulating IgG. In order immune reactions in the oral cavity to be initiated, the antigen should go through the barrier of epithelium.

Importance of Immune Reactions in the Oral Cavity

- Protection from the microbial colonization, adherence and infiltration

- Removal of damaged, infected or necrotic cells and tissues

- Distinction of "self" from the foreign

- Prevention of sensitization of adjacent regions

Factors Playing Important Role in the Immune Reactions of Oral Cavity

- Secretory immunoglobulin A

- Cells of lymphatic tissue of the oral mucosa

Secretory IgA

Production: 3 g sIgA per day

Isotypes: A1 and A2. A2 is derived from plasma cells.

It is constituted by secretory region and Jchain

Secretory region: It has a molecular weight of 80,000. It is composed and secreted by oral epithelial cells.

J chain:

Molecular weight: 15,600 kDa

It is related with immunoglobulin polymerism

It is composed by plasma cells

It determines the degree of bacterial adherence

Lymphatic Tissue of the Oral Mucosa

It includes bone marrow cells, thymus and spleen cells, as well as cells from regional lymph nodes.

Cells of Lymphatic Tissue of Oral Mucosa

Antigen presenting cells (Langerhans cells and macrophages)

Endoepithelial lymphocytes

Lymphocytes of connective tissue

Plasma cells that produce sIgA

Cells that have been antigenically irritated

Ways of Antigen Recognition

In oral cavity and in all stratified squamous epithelia

antigen recognition is based on Langerhans cells

Langerhans cells transport and present the antigen in the nearest lymphatic focus

Antigen Passage Through the Epithelium

- Transport is an active process facilitated by Langerhans cells

- Obstacles are the cellular junctions, sIgA, mucins etc

- The peptides and the macromolecules go through the epithelium with more difficulty

Adherence of Antigen on the Antigen-Presenting Cell

- The mechanism is unclear

- Adherence requires endocytotic mechanisms

- The "adhesive" substances create immune reactions

- The adherence implicates a very wide spectrum of antigens

Antigen Recognition

After the antigenic stimulation, lymphocytes migrate towards oral mucosa.

Lymphocytes that have not been antigenically stimulated do not have clear preferences as to the place of migration.

In the contrary, lymphocytes that have been antigenically irritated present clear preferences and precise knowledge of the place of migration.

Permeability of Oral Mucosa

Oral mucosa does not allow the passage of big particles (e.g. microorganisms). It only allows the passage of molecules and ions.

The passage routes of various structures via the epithelium are:

- The intercellular spaces

Through the cells

An important factor determining the speed of passage of a substance through the epithelium is his solubility in water or in lipids.

The fat-soluble substances go through the epithelium rapidly, entering easily in the lipid-rich cellular membranes.

The belief that substances pass through the nonkeratinized epithelium more rapidly is wrong. The barriers influencing the passage of substances are same in all epithelial types.

A particular region of oral epithelium regarding its permeability is the gingival attached epithelium. In this region, epithelium is particularly permeable for a big number of bacteria and bacterial microbial toxins.

It is not known if the increased penetrability:

is due to structure peculiarities of attached epithelium or

it is a result of bacterial plaque.

Connective tissue is more permeable compared with epithelium. It does not only allow passage of very big molecules.

SENSORY FUNCTIONS

The sensory functions performed by oral mucosa are the senses of touch, gustation, pain, perception of temperature and movement.

Sense of Touch-Mechanoreceptors

The sense of touch is served by the presence of mechanoreceptors of the oral mucosa.

Mechanoreceptors, as their name imply are receptors that correspond in mechanic irritations.

Mechanoreceptors in the orofacial region serve two functions:

➢   They transmit to the brain the sense of food texture

➢   They supply the sensory feedback which is essential for the control of kinetic functions of the orofacial region

As for their second function, mechanoreceptors provide to the nervous system continuous information, regarding the position of food and tongue and the creation of bolus. This information leads to the avoidance of accidental bite and to the protection of tongue and buccal mucosa [2, 3].

Periodontal ligament, a structure that surrounds and attaches teeth in their alveoles, is rich in mechanoreceptors. These mechanoreceptors are stimulated from occlusal forces or by forces beared by the tongue and they provide precious information for the control of kinetic functions of the orofacial region.

Classification of Mechanoreceptors

The classification of mechanoreceptors is based on their neurophysiological response to certain stimuli. Their response is evaluated according:

➢   The behavior during the application and removal of an irritant agent, which is called dynamic phase of irritation

➢   The behavior at the duration of continuous action of an irritant factor, that is named static

phase of irritation. Mechanoreceptors that create potentials solely during the dynamic phase of irritation are known as *rapidly adapting* mechanoreceptors. Mechanoreceptors creating potentials both in the dynamic and static phase are the *slowly* adapting mechanoreceptors. Both of these categories of mechanoreceptors are further subdivided according to their functional characteristics into:

➢   Type I, that have short receptive fields and

➢   Type II, that have longer receptive fields

Types of Mechanoreceptors

<u>*Meissner Corpuscles*</u>

Meissner corpuscles belong to the category of rapidly adapting mechanoreceptors. They are encapsulated unmyelinated nerve endings, which consist of flattened supportive cells arranged as horizontal lamellae surrounded by a connective tissue capsule. The corpuscle is between 30-140 μm in length and 40-60 μm in diameter. They are usually found in the connective tissue papillae and they are linked with collagen fibers with the basement membrane. Several neural fibers enter into these corpuscles and terminate as nerve endings.

<u>*Merkel Cells*</u>

Merkel cells belong to the category of type 1 slowly adapting mechanoreceptors. They are dendritic in shape. The endings of their cytoplasmic projections are discoid. They are located in the basal layer of oral epithelium and they are connected with the adjacent epithelial parts with desmosomes. The origin of Merkel cells is still controversial. Evidence from skin graft experiments in birds implies that they are neural crest derived, while experiments in mammals generally point to an epidermal origin. Most often, they are associated with sensory nerve endings, when they are known as Merkel nerve endings (also called a Merkel cell-neurite complex).

Ruffini's Corpuscles

Ruffini's corpuscles are considered as type 2 slowly adapting mechanoreceptors. They are spindle-shaped receptors, sensitive to tissue stretch, and contribute to the kinesthetic sense and control of tissue position and movement. They consist of an ovoid capsule within which the sensory fiber ends with numerous collateral knobs.

Paccinian corpuscles Paccinian corpuscles are larger and fewer in number than both Merkel cells and Meissner's corpuscles. They are oval shaped and approximately 1 mm in length. Concentric layers of Schwann cells surrounding a central single afferent unmyelinated nerve ending constitute them. Paccinian corpuscles detect gross pressure changes and vibrations. They are characterized as type 2 rapidly adapting mechanoreceptors.

Functional Characteristics of Oral Mucosa Mechanoreceptors

The receptive field of type 1 rapidly and slowly adapting mechanoreceptors is small (3-5mm in diameter). Their sensitivity is high and almost uniform across their receptive field. A significant characteristic of type 1 mechanoreceptors is their capability to respond to stimuli applied to the periphery of their receptive field. In other words, they have the capability to provide information relevant to the texture and the form of the mechanical irritation.

In contrast, the receptive field of type 2 mechanoreceptors is long (up to 8 cm in diameter). The sensitivity of the mechanoreceptor diminishes as the distance from the irritation becomes longer. Type 2 mechanoreceptors respond to vibrational stimuli between 100-300 Hz. Another characteristic of type 2 mechanoreceptors is that they respond to stretching or contraction of the oral mucosa.

Mechanoreceptors of Periodontal Tissues

Mechanoreceptors of periodontal ligament are similar with Ruffini's corpuscles. Functionally they belong both to rapidly adapting mechanoreceptors and to slowly adapting mechanoreceptors [4]. In humans, the predominant type is slowly adapting mechanoreceptors. The innervation of periodontal mechanoreceptors is achieved with afferent neural fibers that have their cellular bodies in the trigeminal ganglion or in the mesenchephalic nucleus. Mechanoreceptors that are related with trigeminal ganglion are located to the middle part of the tooth, while those that are related with mesenchephalic nucleus are located to the apical part of the tooth.

Mechanical irritations applied to the teeth cause tension of the periodontal ligament and subsequent stimulation of periodontal mechanoreceptors. Rapidly adapting mechanoreceptors respond to movements of the teeth, while the response of slowly adapting mechanoreceptors depends on the intensity of the mechanical stimulus. Both rapidly and slowly adapting mechanoreceptors respond according to the direction of stimulus.

Certain periodontal mechanoreceptors do not have sensitivity related to the arrangement of collagen fibers in periodontal tissues.

Perception of Temperature Thermoreceptors

The perception of temperature in the oral cavity is mandatory for the qualitative evaluation of food. Certain foods should be cooked and served in different temperatures in order to be delicious. Oral mucosa does not have uniform sensitivity in temperature. It has instead distinct areas of sensitivity to warmth and cold. Thermoreceptors respond to food temperature and send the appropriate information to the central nervous system. Depending on their response to warmth and cold, thermoreceptors are classified into warmth and cold receptors. Regardless of the initial temperature, a warmth receptor responds to a sudden increase of the temperature, while it provisionally suspends its activity to a decrease of temperature [5]. Exactly the opposite occurs with cold receptors.

Differences between warmth and cold receptors are observed during the period of constant temperatures or during the period of static response frequency. Thermoreceptors always react actively to the changes of the temperature in the oral cavity. They have the capacity to stimulate the reflexes of sweating and tremor. Temperatures likely to damage the oral cavity are sensed by sub-categories of nociceptors that may respond to noxious cold, noxious heat or more than one noxious stimulus modality (i.e. they are polymodal).

Cold receptors are found in rather superficial regions of skin and oral mucosa. It has been estimated that cold receptors are found 0.18 mm under the surface of the skin, while warm receptors are located in a deeper region (0.22 mm).

In the mammalian peripheral nervous system, warmth receptors are believed to be unmyelinated C-fibers (low conduction velocity), while those responding to cold, have thin myelinated A delta fibers (faster conduction velocity). The receptive field of thermoreceptors is short (less than 1 mm^2). Hypothalamus is involved in thermoregulation. Thermoreceptors provide feed-forward responses to changes in body temperature. Unlike mechanoreceptors, which are silent in the absence of tactile stimuli, thermoreceptors fire action potentials continuously at low rates when the skin temperature is set at its normal value of 34^0C. Cold and warmth receptors differ in the range of static temperatures to which they respond. Cold receptors respond to steady-state temperatures of 5-40^0C. Warmth receptors are active at steady temperatures of 29-45^0C. At normal skin temperature of 34^0C cold receptors are more active than warmth receptors.

Transduction Mechanisms of Thermoreceptors

The adequate stimulus for a warmth receptor is warming, which results in an increase in their action potential discharge rate. Cooling results in a decrease in warm receptor discharge rate.

Transduction mechanisms of thermoreceptors gained considerable attention after the identification and cloning of the Transient Receptor Potential (TRP) family of proteins. Transient receptor potential or TRP channels are a family of ion channels that are relatively non-selectively permeable to cations, including sodium, calcium and magnesium [6].

Temperature changes modulate the activity of the Na^+/K^+-ATPase pump. The Na^+/K^+-ATPase is a P-type pump that extrudes Na^+ ions in exchange for K^+ ions for each hydrolytic cleavage of ATP. This results in a movement of positive charge out of the cell, i.e. a hyperpolarizing current.

Proprioception

Proprioception is the sense of the relative position of neighboring parts of the body. Proprioception is a distinct sensory modality that provides feedback solely on the status of the body internally.

Kinesthesia is another term that is often used interchangeably with proprioception, though use of the term "kinesthesia" can place a greater emphasis on motion.

In the orofacial region, proprioception mainly concerns the sense of movement and the position of mandible and the tongue.

The initiation of proprioception is the activation of specific receptors for this form of perception termed "proprioceptors". The proprioceptive sense is believed to be composed of information from sensory neurons located in the inner ear (motion and orientation) and in the stretch receptors located in the muscles and the joint-supporting ligaments. The main proprioceptors of the orofacial region are muscle spindles, Golgi tendon organ and joint receptors.

Muscle Spindles

Muscle spindles are sensory receptors within a muscle, which primarily detect changes in the length of this muscle. They convey length information to the central nervous system via sensory neurons. This information can be processed by the brain to determine the position of body parts.

Muscle spindles do not only play primary role in proprioception, but also assist considerably in the sensory feedback, which is essential for the movements of the mandible [7].

They are spindle-shaped, encapsulated by connective tissue and are aligned parallel to extrafusal muscle fibers.

The muscle spindles have both sensory and motor components. Sensory nerve fibers spiral around and terminate on the central portions of the intrafusal muscle fibers, providing the sensory component of the structure via stretch-sensitive ion-channels of the axons. The motor component is provided by gamma motoneurons and to a lesser extent by beta motoneurons. Gamma and beta motoneurons are termed fusimotor neurons, because they activate the intrafusal muscle fibers. Gamma motoneurons are subdivided into three categories; $\gamma 1$, $\gamma 2$ and $\gamma 3$ [8].

The muscle fibers extend from one to the other pole of the receptor. They are subdivided into two morphological types; nuclear-bag and nuclear-chain. Both of them have the capability of muscular contraction.

Golgi Tendon Organ

Golgi tendon organ is constituted from a bundle of spindle-shaped small tendons, which are innervated by afferent neuronal fibers of big diameter. Fifty or even more organelles of this type are located in the regions where the muscle is connected with his tendon. Activation of Golgi tendon organ is provided by alpha motoneurons. Golgi tendon organs are very sensitive receptors responding to forces starting from only 30mgr.

Joint Receptors

Joints contain numerous slowly adapting mechanoreceptors, which react to the stretching of ligaments and joint capsules.

The receptors located in ligaments are similar with Golgi tendon organs, while the receptors of the capsules are identical with Ruffini's corpuscles.

The role of joint receptors is most likely related with torsion and not with kinesthesia. Therefore, in most instances their role is protective. A classic example is a soccer player who wants to kick the ball but fails to come into contact. In this case, knee joints receptors instantly react protecting the knee from overstretching.

Proprioceptors in the Orofacial Region

The joints contain many slow adapting mechanoreceptors, which react to stretching of the ligaments and joint capsules.

Muscular receptors are located in:

✓ Masseter

✓ Temporal muscle

✓ Median pterygoid muscle

Golgi tendon organs are found in:

✓ Small numbers into deep layers of masseter and

✓ Temporal muscle

Interfaces of Proprioceptors with the Nervous System

The cellular bodies of the afferent neurons of muscular receptors are located in the mesenchephalic trigeminal nucleus.

The cellular bodies of temporomandibular joint receptors are located in the lateral-posterior region of trigeminal ganglion [9,10].

Pain

Pain can be perceptible from every tissue of the orofacial region including the teeth even if enamel is not sensitive and a direct excitation of dentin should exist.

Pain receptors do not have any distinct morphological characteristics; they simply appear as pain endings, which are similar with those of touch, warmth or cold. There is no acknowledged definition of noxious stimuli. It is clear that pain does not constitute an overexcitation of a certain sense, such as touch or temperature; it seems to be related with a tissue injury at cellular level. Physiologists, who study the reactions of animals to noxious stimuli, do not use the term pain because it rather contains a sentimental element. The term noxious is used instead.

Products of inflammation or tissue destruction, such as hydrogen ions, potassium ions, certain prostaglandins, polypeptides, histamine and serotonin, stimulate neurons participating in noxious perception.

Two types of neuronal fibers participate in the transmission of signals that lead to perception of pain:

✓ Myelinated fibers Aδ, 2.5µm in diameter, speed of transmission 12-30 m/s

✓ Unmyelinated C fibers, 0.4-1.2 µm in diameter, speed of transmission 0,5-2m/s

Aδ fibers can transmit information from pain receptors or from mechanoreceptors. C fibers are characterized as proprioceptive receptors and are capable of transmitting a number of different impulses. Several neurotransmitters, such as substance P, glutaminic acid and neurokine A participate in the signal transmission process both for Aδ and C fibers. These two types of fibers transmit different senses of pain. Aδ fibers are related with an acute, localized sense, which is usually a result of a mechanical injury. This pain is called primary pain. C fibers are associated with a widespread, dull pain, which usually follows primary pain or may rise because of various stimuli. The repeated stimulate on of Aδ and C fibers leads to hyperalgesia. Hyperalgesia is an increased sensitivity to pain, which may be caused by damage to nociceptors or peripheral nerves. Hyperalgesia is subdivided into primary and secondary. Primary hyperalgesia describes pain sensitivity that occurs directly in the damaged tissues. Secondary hyperalgesia describes pain sensitivity that occurs in surrounding undamaged tissues. Example of hyperalgesia is trigeminal neuralgia. In trigeminal neuralgia even the slightest stimulation of the trigger zones, causes intense and long lasting pain, which does not correspond to the common analgesic treatments. Neuronal fibers are headed from the proprioceptive final endings, through the spinal bundle of the trigeminal nerve, to the median nucleus of spinal bundle. These fibers are located posteriorly and internally of the maxillary nerve, which is found posteriorly of the ophthalmic nerve neurons. Spinal bundle of the trigeminal nerve is an extension of the posterior gelatinosa matter of the spinal cord. The gray matter of medulla oblongata is divided in eight zones, which are analogous with those decribed in the spinal cord literature. The main neurons that end into zone I are unmyelinated C and a few Aδ and Aβ fibers. C fibers are proprioceptive. They are distributed in the region of nucleus caudalis and they make synapses with neurons passing through the spinal cord and the reticulothalamic way. Although these receptors are proprioceptive, some of them respond in very low mechanical stimulation. They have short receptive fields. Zones II and III are layers of the posterior gelatinosa matter. They receive signals from large myelinated fibers, such as from mechanoreceptors and from Aδ fibers with very short receptive fields. These zones, particularly zones III and IV, have numerous intermediate stimulatory or inhibitory neurons. Intermediate neurons, especially the inhibitory, are linked with all other zones. Zones IV-VI receive signals from proprioceptors that have large receptive fields. Zone V additionally receives signals from touch and pressure receptors via Aβ fibers and from temperature receptors via Aδ fibers. In this zone, many neurons have large receptive fields. This results in an ambiguous localization of the stimulated area. Zones VI-VIII constitute a part of the reticular activating system whose sensory function is considered non specific. Although the fibers from this region can be projected in the posterior celiac nucleus of thalamus and in the somatosensory cortex, many times they are connected via hypothalamus with regions of the cortex enabling to the perceived senses to acquire an emotional coherence. The cells of zone IV and V in the spinal cord are believed to transmit the information of pain according to the theory of gate control. Theory of gate control was an effort to explain why thesimultaneous stimulation of other proprioceptors can inhibit the perception of pain. If the impulses in the proprioceptive neurons could reach to the cortex, then the "gates" of pain would open and pain would be perceivable. If the transmission in the synapses of the posterior gelatinosa matter was intercepted by inhibitory impulses in intermediate neurons connected with large sensory afferent fibers, then the "gates" of pain would stay closed.

This theoretically explains why the application of pressure in an area of pain, even clenching of affected tooth, can temporarily relieve the pain. Counter-irritants function with the same way. Gate control theory also gives possible explanations for some forms of acupuncture. A weak point of gate control theory is its simplicity regarding the region of pain inhibition. Today it is clear that proprioceptive neurons have synapses in many levels and that inhibition is a result of connections with neurons of the same or other levels of brain. A modification of the theories regarding pain perception was made after the discovery of endorphins and the associated enchephalins. The identification of morphine receptors lead to the discovery of a group of two peptides; endorphins with 15 and 31 aminoacids respectively, which are produced in the brain and the pituitary gland. Further investigation revealed the existence of two smaller peptides with five aminoacids as active transmitters. These peptides are produced in situations in which the perception of pain was smaller than the expected according to the intensity of stimulation. More recently, dynorphines, a group of bigger peptides was discovered. The release of enchephalins reduces or inhibits the release of substance P. Substance P is a neurotransmitter which is often associated with the routes of pain transmission. Higher concentrations of substance P in the nervous system are found in the trigeminal spinal nucleus. Experiments in animals have shown that nucleus caudalis actively transmits pain impulses in the presence of naloxone. Naloxone blocks morphine receptors. Electrical stimulation of certain areas, such as reticular formation, major suture nucleus, lower central suture nucleus and gray matter around cerebral aqueduct, causes analgesia in the area that trigeminal nerve is distributed, without influencing the transmission from other afferent neurons.

There are also other connections between major suture nucleus and trigeminal fibers using serotonin as a neurotransmitter instead of enchephalins. These connections are not inhibitory.Endorphins are derivatives of a single gene while enchephalins are encoded by two genes; one is for met-enchephalin and the second is for leu-enchephalin. The second gene also encodes dynorphines, another group of peptides with analgesic properties. Enchephalins have a very short half-life and they have not found to be effective in pain inhibition. However, the idea of sensory nerve stimulation for pain inhibition and induction of analgesia during dental operations has been applied with transcutaneous electrical nerve stimulation (TENS). While part of pain perception derives from the transmission of impulses in the somatosensory cortex, there is a part originating from impulses in the fibers of reticular system. These impulses pass through hypothalamus and limbic cortex obtaining an emotional significance, which is recognized as the unpleasant nature of pain. Pain differs from the other senses by possessing this strong emotional feature, which may be pleasant or unpleasant. Some patients may suck or move a tooth and they may feel satisfaction for the affordable sense of stabbing pain. Apart from the afferent routes in the brainstem and limbic system there are abductory fibers which can inhibit the proprioceptive transmission. Psychological agents significantly influence the perception of pain. Fear and anxiety lower the threshold of pain. Enthusiasm and relaxation may raise the threshold of pain. Relaxing music or even a mixture of high frequencies known as "white sound" is used in the so-called echo analgesia.

Gustation

Taste (or, more formally, gustation) is a form of direct chemoreception. It refers to the ability to detect the flavor of substances such as food, certain minerals, and poisons. In humans and many other vertebrate animals, the sense of taste collaborates with the less direct sense of smell, in the brain's perception of flavor. Even bacteria possess receptors sensitive to chemical substances. For the perception of gustation essential are the presence of taste buds and the presence of afferent neurons towards brainstem and thalamus. There are five basic tastes: bitter, salty, sour, sweet, and umami (described as savory, meaty, or brothy). The basic tastes are only one component that contributes to the sensation of food in the mouth—other factors include the food's smell, detected by the olfactory epithelium of the nose, its texture, detected by mechanoreceptors, and its temperature, detected by thermoreceptors [11]. Taste and smell are subsumed under the term "flavor".

Taste Buds

Taste buds in most mammals are located in oropharynx and larynx. A big number of taste buds are located on the dorsal and lateral surface of the tongue, on certain mucosal projections that are termed papillae. There are four types of papillae; fungiform, filiform, circumvallate and foliate. Foliate papillae in humans are vestigial. Filiform are numerous and constitute the majority of all papillae in the oral cavity. However, they lack taste buds and they do not participate in the function of gestation.

Fungiform papillae are fewer. They are located in the anterior two thirds of the dorsal surface of the tongue and bear one or more test buds in their upper part.

Circumvallate papillae are located at the borderline between oral and pharyngeal part of the tongue, in front of the sulcus terminalis.

In humans, there are 8-12 circumvallate papillae on the dorsal surface of the tongue, in front of the foramen cecum and sulcus terminalis, forming the so-called gustatory lambda. Every circumvallate papilla consists of a projection of mucous membrane attached to the bottom of a circular depression of the mucous membrane. The margin of the depression is elevated to form a wall (vallum). Between vallum and the papilla there is a circular sulcus termed the fossa. The papilla has a form of a truncated cone, the narrower end being directed downward and attached to the tongue and the wider end projecting above the surface of the tongue and being covered by stratified squamous epithelium.

In the lateral surfaces of the tongue there are foldings named filiform papillae. Taste buds are located within their epithelium.

In neonates, all papillae bear taste buds. The location of taste buds plays has been linked with their specificity for recognition of various flavors. Taste buds located at the tip of the tongue are responsible for the sweet flavor, taste buds at the lateral surfaces of the tongue identify the bitter and salty flavor, while taste buds located at the posterior third of the tongue and on palate identify bitter and sour flavor. Other regions of the oral mucosa hosting taste buds are soft palate, the posterior part of epiglottis and pharynx and glossopalatal foldings.

Structure of Taste Buds

Every taste bud is constituted of 30-60 fusiform epithelial cells that extend from basement membrane up to the free surface of the epithelium. These cells have a life span of 10-11 days and are surrounded by other epithelial cells that are constantly renewed. Taste buds communicate with the external environment through a narrow tube, which is named gustatory duct.

The endings of gustatory nerve enter into taste buds, they ramify and finally are connected with epithelial cells.

Electron microscopy observations have revealed that four types of epithelial cells exist in taste buds. Type I (dark cells) constitutes 60% of all epithelial cells in the taste bud. It is characterized by the presence of cells with pycnotic vesicles in their cytoplasm and toothy-shaped nucleus. Type II (luminous cells) is characterized by electron-lucent cytoplasm with large round or oval nuclei. Type III resembles type II. One difference is the projections that are extended into the gustatory duct. Finally, type IV consists of cells that do not reach gustatory duct and are named basal cells.

The initial contact between gustatory stimulus and taste bud is performed in the gustatory duct region.

Dynamic Properties of Taste Buds

The cells of taste buds as well as their surrounding epithelial cells are constantly renewed. Their life span is 10-11 days. Various studies have shown that these cells migrate from the periphery to the taste bud center. This migration raises some questions regarding the way that epithelial cells are connected with gustatory nerve endings. One possibility is the taste bud cells to have the capacity of rapidly changing nerve connections and another possibility is to maintain the same neural fiber until their death.

Another dynamic property of taste buds is their capacity for rapid regeneration. This capacity is probably linked with the presence of gustatory nerves. It has been shown that in regions where gustatory nerves have been surgically removed a simultaneous disappearance of taste buds takes place.

Mechanisms in the Taste Buds

The first efforts to understand the nature of the receptors on the taste buds, which react with the gustatory stimulus begun in the early 60's when for the first time a catheterization of gustatory ducts was attempted.

However, the most significant advances in this field were achieved during the last years after the study of the biochemical characteristics and currents in the cell membranes of taste buds.

Several mechanisms have been implicated in the transduction of gustatory stimulus. The most important is the ion channel mechanism. According to this mechanism, the epithelial cells of taste buds bear ion channels on their cell surfaces. The flow of cations opens these channels that results in depolarization or hyperpolarization of cells [12]. Very few things are today known about gustatory receptors on the cell surfaces of taste buds. One known fact is the adjacency of taste bud receptors with ion channels. Every cell of taste buds reacts to more than one gustatory stimuli; sweet, sour, salty and bitter.

Cerebral Centers of Gustation

The transmission of gustatory information to the brain is achieved with the afferent gustatory fibers of facial, glossopharyngeal and vagus nerve, which send the chemosensory information to the solitary nucleus of brainstem. The gustatory nucleus is localized at the anterior part of solitary nucleus, while its caudal part is responsible for the control of many somatosensory functions. After brainstem, gustatory stimulus reaches thalamus and finally cerebral cortex [13,14].

Changes of Taste Buds with Age

Taste buds appear very early in the human tongue. They initially appear during the 7th or 8th week of gestation and their final configuration ends after birth.

Studies on neonates' behavior have shown that during birth there is a gustatory capability of a certain degree especially to the salty flavor. This probably means that certain parameters of gustation are innate and do not require any experience. It also has been suggested that these innate perceptions of taste is possible to be altered after an intense and persistent gustatory experience. In the other flavors, every neonate reacts differently [15].

The aging process of the organism does not influence significantly the gustatory system. In several studies, the reduction of gustatory capability in elderly individuals was found very small and statistically not significant.

The Role of Saliva in Gustation

The presence of saliva is essential for the gustatory process. Reduction of saliva results in significant reduction of gustatory capability. Saliva does not only act as a solvent of food. It also helps for food transportation to taste buds. It also acts as a buffering solution and plays a significant role in the transduction of the gustatory stimulus.

The role of saliva in transportation of gustatory stimulus: a saliva layer permanently coats taste buds. Taste buds of fungiform and filiform papillae are always coated by saliva that is secreted by all salivary glands. Taste buds of circumscribed and filiform papillae are saturated with saliva from Von Ebner's glands, while the remaining taste buds of palate and pharynx are saturated with saliva from minor salivary glands.

The transportation of gustatory stimuli to the taste buds during the intake of solid or liquid food is achieved with coordinated movements of the muscles moving the mandible, tongue and face.

The Role of Saliva in the Transduction of Gustatory Stimulus

One of the organic components of saliva is the rich in proteins prolines. These proteins are linked with the capability of bitter flavor perception. They are believed to act as molecule transporters of substances with bitter flavor.

Recently it has been shown that Von Ebners' glands secrete a protein similar with those that block smells in the nasal mucosa. This protein is not secreted by other salivary glands and it is considered essential for the transportation of the lipophilic stimuli in taste buds. It has been also linked with the perception of sweet flavor, since many substances with sweet flavor are lipophilic [16].

Effect of Xerostomia in Taste Perception

Observations on individuals that had received radiotherapy of the orofacial region have shown that xerostomia negatively affects gustatory perception. Surgical removal of the salivary glands or administration of parasympatholytic substances in experimental animals, have also confirmed the negative effect of xerostomia in gestation. The reduced gustatory capability is probably caused by structural alterations in taste buds, which are surrounded by inflammatory cells and bacteria.

Clinical Disturbances of Taste

Full loss of gustatory capability is termed ageusia, while the partial loss is termed hypogeusia. Other clinical disturbances of taste are dysgeusia and parosmia, which are characterized by a chronic gustatory perception without the presence of a gustatory stimulus [17,18].

Very often, the evaluation of a patient complaining for gustatory disturbances is difficult because taste perception is also configurated by other parameters such as smell, temperature of food and touch.

Factors causing gustatory disturbances are:

- ✓ Vitamin A deficiency. Vitamin A deficiency leads to hyperkeratosis of the tongue mucosa, which results in obstruction of the gustatory duct of taste buds
- ✓ Epilepsy. Gustatory disturbances have been reported in patients with epilepsy.
- ✓ Familial dysautonomia. This pathologic condition frequently occurs in Jewish children. Among other signs, it is characterized by atrophy of tongue mucosa with less papillae and taste buds.
- ✓ Radiotherapy of the orofacial region. Besides other catastrophic effects it destroys taste buds.
- ✓ Malignant neoplasms. They may cause gustatory disturbances that lead in anorexia and in weight loss. The pathogenetic mechanism in these cases is multifactorial.
- ✓ Medications. Many drugs may alter the gustatory perception. Some of them acting in the brain have a central effect in taste, while other alter gestation by being secreted in saliva. An example of a drug secreted in saliva and causing hypogeusia is d-penicillamine Zinc. Zinc deficiency may cause gustatory disturbances.
- ✓ Burning mouth syndrome. Gustatory disturbances can be seen in patients with burning mouth syndrome. Pathogenetic mechanism in these cases is usually multifactorial.

Composition and Secretion of Various Substances

Secretion of Saliva

Saliva is an important component of the oral cavity. Pure saliva is a colorless, odorless and opaque liquid of special weight 1.002-1.012 and pH 6.7-7.4.

It is mainly composed by water and many solid components. Organic and inorganic substances mainly constitute solid components.

Saliva performs many functions. Most important are:

- ✓ Protection of oral mucosa from masticatory frictions
- ✓ Helps in digestion with its various enzymes
- ✓ Helps in the formation of bolus
- ✓ Antibacterial, antifungal and immunologic protection
- ✓ It has buffering capacity
- ✓ Participates in the excretion of various metabolic products
- ✓ Protects teeth from caries
- ✓ Contains growth factors and other regulatory peptides
- ✓ Helps to gestation, cleaning taste buds
- ✓ Helps to speech

Secretion of saliva is continuous 24 hours a day with some fluctuations. The quantity that is daily produced from all salivary glands is 500-750 ml. It is estimated that major salivary glands produce the 90% of the total quantity of saliva, while the remaining 10% is produced from the minor salivary glands, which are spread in many regions of the oral mucosa [19].

Structure of Salivary Glands

Every salivary gland consists of three parts; acinar, duct system and intermediate or supportive tissue. Acinar part is composed of acini, which are subdivided into mucous, serous and mixed. Mucous acini are comprised of large triangular cells with vacuolar cytoplasm. Mucous cells excrete their secretion into the lumen, in the middle of acini and into the secretory capillaries. Serous cells are fewer and have a pyramoid form. Similarly, serous cells excrete their secretion into the lumen and into the secretory capillaries. In the periphery of acini, there are myoepithelial cells. Myoepithelial cells or basket cells lie between the basement membrane and the plasma membrane of the secretory cells. They are also found in the proximal part of the duct system. Myoepithelial cells possess many actin-containing microfilaments, which squeeze on the secretory cells and move their products toward the excretory ducts. Mixed acini are composed both of mucous and serous cells. There are three types of ducts in the salivary glands: intercalated, striated and excretory ducts. Both intercalated and secretory ducts are found within the parenchyma of the gland and are therefore intralobular ducts. Intercalated ducts are slender ducts continuous with the terminal acini, and lined with flat, spindle-shaped cells. They secrete bicarbonate ion into and absorb chloride ion from the acinar product. Striated ducts resorb sodium and secrete potassium. As they approach the excretory ducts, their diameter may exceedthat of the acini. The largest ducts are the excretory ducts. They are found in the connective tissue septa, and are therefore interlobular ducts. Excretory ducts do not change the secretory product. The system of ducts in the minor salivary glands is different. Intercalated and striated ducts are usually absent. Only secretory ducts are found. Lobes and lobules are composed of loose connective tissue, who has a rich vascular, lymphatic and neural network.

Composition of Saliva

Saliva is a solution consisting 99% of water and 1% of organic and inorganic constituents. Compared to serum is considered hypotonic solution.

Saliva components are the following:

- ■ Derivatives from salivary glands
  - - Water, proteins, electrolytes, small organic molecules

- Blood and blood derivatives
    - Red and white cells gingival crevicular fluid and inflammatory cells
- Exogenous substances
    - Food remains, toothpastes and mouthwashes
- Other liquids
    - Bronchial and nasal secretions
- Cells
    - Epithelial cells
- Micro-organisms

<u>Inorganic components</u>: The main salivary cations are sodium and potassium. As for the anions most important are chlorides and bicarbonates. Other salivary electrolytes are magnesium, calcium, phosphates, iodine, copper, fluorine, sulfuric and thiocyanate salts.

<u>Organic components</u>: The main organic salivary components include mucin 1 and 2, histatine, statherins, various glycoproteins, amylase, lipase, carbonic dehydrases, lactoferrin, lysozyme, peroxidase system and secretory immunoglobulin A.

The most significant functions of mucin are:

- Coating of tissues
    - Coating of hard and soft palate
    - Mainly participates in acquired salivary pellicle formation
    - Keeps antibacterial agents on the mucosal surfaces
- Lubricative action
    - It is aligned with the flux direction (characteristic of the asymmetric molecules)
    - Increases the lubricative capacity of saliva, increasing the coherence of coatings
    - Coherence of coatings is an important factor for frictions reduction

Histatines are a group of proteins rich in histidine and they are potential inhibitors of *Candida albicans.*

Statherins intercept the sedimentation of supersaturated phosphoric salts in saliva, contributing to the good enamel coherence.

Rich in praline glycoproteins are subdivided into alkaline and acid. Alkaline glycoproteins block the lipids and contribute to their absorption through the cell membranes, while acid glycoproteins contribute to calcium attachment on the dental surfaces. Rich in proline glycoproteins inhibit the formation of phosphate calcium crystals and are found in enamel pellicle.

Amylase hydrolizes the a(1-4) bonds of amylum contributing to the initial process of digestion. Amylase also participates in bacterial attachment on the dental surfaces.

Lipase is secreted from Von Ebner's glands of the tongue. It participates in the first phase of fat digestion and hydrolizes triglycerides. It is considered significant factor for digestion of milk fat in neonates.

Lactoferrin is a salivary antibacterial factor that blocks ferrum used for bacterial metabolism. Certain microorganisms (i.e. *E.coli)* adapt to this condition secreting enterochelines, which block ferrum more efficiently than lactoferrin. Bacteria reabsorb rich in ferrum enterochelines.

Lactoferrin with or without ferrum is broken up by certain bacterial proteases. In non-bound condition, it has antibacterial action.

Lysozyme is an antibacterial agent found in various organs and secretions.

Salivary lysozyme originates:

✓   From salivary glands

✓   From phagocytes

✓   From gingival crevicular fluid

It has the capability of hydrolyzing chemical bonds of bacterial polysaccharides. Gram-negative bacteria are more resistant in lysozyme action because their bacterial wall is tough. Salivary peroxidase system include sialoperoxidase, myeloperoxidase, H_2O_2. and thiocyanate salts which after the peroxidase action and are transformed into hypothiocyanate salts. Sialoperoxidase is produced in parotid gland acini. It is also present in submandibular gland saliva. It is absorbed by enamel, bacteria and microbial plaque. Myeloperoxidase is produced by white cells. It is found in the gingival crevicular fluid.

The antimicrobial capability of hypothiocyanates salts is based on their capacity to oxidize sulphydrylic bonds, to inhibit glucose uptake and transportation of aminoacids, to destroy cell membranes and to interrupt electrochemical changes.

Other organic substances, which are found in saliva but are not secreted by salivary glands are secretory immunoglobulin A (s-IgA), carbohydrates, aminoacids, uric acid, creatinine, vitamins, alkaline and acid phosphatase, kallikrein, cholinesterase, hyalouronidase etc. Isohaemagglutinins A, B and O may also be present [20].

Factors Affecting the Composition of Saliva

The composition of saliva is mainly influenced by three factors:

✓   Type of salivary gland

✓   Type and intensity of stimulus

✓   The hour of day and night

One of the parameters of salivary secretion that has been extensively studied is the effect of salivary flow on salivary composition. If salivary flow is studied during day and night without the interference of any other apparent factor (i.e. food intake), it is obvious that certain circadian rhythms exist. This finding implies that salivary glands produce fluctuating amounts of saliva all over day and night. Increase of salivary flow is observed in periods of food intake or during periods of expectation for food intake and is always combined with alterations of salivary components. Concentration of certain salivary components, such as sodium, may be increased with the increase of salivary flow. In contrast, potassium concentration is decreased as salivary flow increases. In every salivary gland, salivary flow is under the control of autonomic nervous system. Parasympathetic activity is particularly efficient in the increase of salivary flow, while sympathetic activity is less effective.

Secretion of Water and Electrolytes

The initial saliva produced by acini is secreted into the acinar lumen. Its composition regarding the concentrations of Na+, Cland $HCO_3$is similar with those of serum. In the second phase of salivary secretion, the initial saliva is modified as it passes through secretory duct. Despite the fact that the wall of ducts is not permeable to water, sodium is reabsorbed, while potassium is secreted to the external environment passing through the wall of the secretory duct. When salivary flow is slow, the mechanism of sodium reabsorption is capable to remove the whole sodium from saliva before it reaches to the oral cavity. In contrast, when salivary flow is increased the degree of sodium reabsorption is low and this finally results in increased levels of sodium when saliva reaches the oral cavity. In contrast, when salivary flow is slow potassium is secreted normally, while in increased salivary flow potassium secretion is decreased.

The type of neural stimulation also influences electrolyte secretion. Parasympathetic activity inhibits sodium reabsorption and potassium secretion. This results in production of saliva rich in sodium. In contrast, stimulation of sympathetic system contributes in secretion of saliva rich in proteins.

Secretion of Proteins

The process of protein secretion from salivary glands initially begins with aminoacid uptake, peptide synthesis, glycosylation, condense and exocytosis.

Peptide synthesis and glycosylation are performed in the rough endoplasmic reticulum and in Golgi apparatus. Protein condense initially takes place in Golgi apparatus and is continued in vacuoles and in the secretory granules. Secretory granules are degranularized and then they enter in the process of exocytosis.

Proteins can be secreted in saliva with several ways without the participation of salivary granules. The protracted stimulation of autonomic nervous system contributes to protein secretion without the destruction of secretory granules.

Most of the salivary organic constituents are secreted by acini. However, certain proteins are secreted from the cells of the secretory duct wall. These proteins include several growth factors (i.e. epidermal and nerve growth factor) and peptic enzymes (i.e. ribonuclease and proteinases). Some of these peptides are under hormonal control and are secreted after stimulation of a-adrenergic receptors.

Control of Salivary Secretion

Control from Parasympathetic System

The kinetic-secretory parasympathetic neurons of the salivary glands are located in the salivatory nucleus, which is extended from the anterior pole of the dorsal nucleus of the vagus nerve up to the region of facial nerve in medulla oblongata.

Electrical stimulation of these neurons causes saliva secretion. The cell bodies of parasympathetic neurons have a fusiform shape with two dendritic projections. These projections end in the trigeminal and solitary nucleus. The abductory fibers start from salivatory nucleus and finally end through the cranial nerves in all salivary glands. Parasympathetic innervation of submandibular and hypoglossal gland is performed from intermediate nerve (esthetic branch of facial nerve), while innervation of the parotid gland through the vagus nerve.

Control from the sympathetic system: Salivary glands innervation from sympathetic system is mainly performed from the upper cervical ganglion. The cell bodies of preganglial fibers of the upper cervical ganglion are located at the posterior-intermediate nucleus, which is located at the upper thoracic region of the spinal cord.

Distribution of Neural Fibers in the Salivary Glands

Neural fibers arriving at salivary glands are distributed and interconnected with acini, myoepithelial cells and blood vessels. The connection of nerve endings with the salivary glands is performed with two ways; the first is of sympathetic, while the second is of parasympathetic type. Every neural fiber has the capacity to innervate more than one glandular element (acini, myoepithelial cells). Since every nerve ending contains different types of neurotransmitters, neural stimulation causes complex results in the respective region of the gland.

Acinar Stimulatory Mechanisms for Saliva Secretion

Saliva secretion starts when neurotransmitters are attached on the cell surface receptors of the acinar cells. Acinar cells contain numerous receptors capable of reacting with several neurotransmitters. The vast majority of acinar cells possess cholinergic (muscarinic) receptors. The neurotransmittory substance is acetylcholine, which acts on the cholinergic or muscarinic receptors. Norepinephrine acts as a postganglial sympathetic neurotransmitter.

Recent studies have shown that saliva secretion is not solely related with stimulation of cholinergic receptors. It may be instead co-assisted by the action of certain neuropeptides, such as substance P, vasoactive enteric peptide and calcitonin peptide.

Stimulatory Mechanisms in Myoepithelial Cells

Myoepithelial cells are innervated by sympathetic and parasympathetic nerve fibers. Stimulation of these fibers causes contraction of myoepithelial cells, increase of pressure in the secretory ducts and finally saliva secretion.

The contraction of myoepithelial cells from parasympathetic activity requires participation of cholinergic receptors, while the contraction from sympathetic activity is under the control of a-adrenergic receptors.

Reflexes of Saliva Secretion

The entrance of food in the oral cavity stimulates saliva secretion. This reflex is caused due to the stimulation of the oral mucosa, periodontal ligament and taste buds mechanoreceptors.

Anesthetization of the oral mucosa results in decreased saliva secretion.

Both sympathetic and parasympathetic systems are providing information from the oral cavity to the brainstem region. Abductory neural transmissions travel through the sensory trigeminal, facial and glossopharyngeal nerve fibers and finally arrive at the trigeminal and solitary nucleus.

The afferent to the salivary glands neural transmissions originate from parasympathetic salivatory nucleus and the sympathetic nucleus of the spinal cord.

Secretion of saliva during mastication is more intense at the working side of the mouth.

The sort and the flavor of the food significantly increase salivary secretion. For example, citric acid causes intense salivary secretion. Sucrose in contrast causes increase of salivary amylase whereas its effect on salivary secretion is negligible. Given that increased salivary secretion is affected by parasympathetic system and amylase production is influenced by sympathetic system activity, it is evident that the process of salivary secretion is a result of interactions among mechanoreceptors of the oral mucosa, sympathetic and parasympathetic nuclei that are located in brainstem and the spinal cord.

Functions of Saliva

One of the saliva's main functions is maintenance of good oral hygiene and caries prevention. This is achieved by acid formation limitation caused by bacterial activity. Presence of acids erodes enamel surface and this is the initial stage of caries formation. The most common region where acids are formed is the microbial plaque. Various studies have shown that the dry microbial plaque, which is not exposed to saliva, has lower pH compared to the wet microbial plaque. Saliva's capacity to control microbial plaque's pH is due to its constituents; mainly to bicarbonates. Bicarbonate levels are fluctuating. For example in the resting parotid saliva their concentration is 0.6mEq/L, while after stimulation the concentration is increased to 30mEq/L. Subsequently during the hours of sleep, saliva's capability to control pH is diminished [21].

Aging and Saliva Secretion

Many elderly people often complain for the symptom of xerostomia, for difficulty in swallowing and increased loss of teeth. Based on these observations several older studies had concluded that a decrease in salivary secretion occurs along with aging.

However, recent clinical and experimental data have argued this concept stating that the problem with the older studies was the not detailed evaluation of co-existing pathologic conditions and the non-accurate standardization of salivary flow measurement. Today it is believed that in a healthy elderly person no significant decrease of salivary secretion is observed.

Secretory IgA

IgA in the secretions is different from serum IgA and is termed secretory IgA or sIgA. sIgA's concentration in saliva is 20 mgr/100ml. sIgA consists of κ and λ (light and heavy) chains. Electrophoresis revealed the existence of a small polypeptide, which is different from sIgA's chains. This substance was termed polypeptide J and has a molecular weight of approximately 15.000. Therefore sIgA consists of chain J and a secretory region.

Plasma cells which are located in the connective tissue secrete dimerous sIgA molecules which include one unit of J chain. This molecule is then bonded with the secretory region which is located in the cell membrane of the epithelial cells and the final product is a sIgA molecule.

The mechanisms of sIgA action are:

✓   Inhibition of bacterial attachment or growth on epithelial cells or oral cavity surfaces

✓   Neutralization of viruses and toxins

✓   Elimination of antigens by obstructing antigen entrance and contact with the immune system

Gingival Crevicular Fluid

Gingival crevice fluid (GCF) is a complex mixture of substances derived from serum, leukocytes, and structural cells of the periodontium and oral bacteria

Functions of Gingival Crevicular Fluid

✓   cleans the gingival crevice

✓   contains proteins facilitating epithelial attachment on dental surfaces

✓   it has antibacterial action

Characteristics of the Epithelium of Gingival Crevice

✓   It is coating gingival crevice

✓   It is non keratinized multilayered stratified epithelium

✓   There is no granular layer

✓   There are no epithelial rete ridges

✓   There are no Merkel cells

Gingival Crevicular Fluid is a Mixture Consisting of

✓   serum derivatives (white cells, proteins)

✓   cells of periodontal tissue

✓   micro-organisms

Most Significant Constituents of Gingival Crevicular Fluid are

✓   antibodies

✓   enzymes

✓   factors of tissue break down

Antibodies originate from molecule synthesis in local as well as in systemic level. They reflect the colonization of gingival crevice by bacteria. Proteolytic enzymes are frequently found in gingival crevicular fluid. They originate from epithelial or connective tissue cells. The most frequent proteolytic enzymes are metalloproteinases, which are responsible for the break down of periodontal tissues. Analysis of gingival crevicular fluid may give a view of an existing periodontal disease.

REFERENCES

[1]   Murata K, Baldwin WM. Mechanisms of complement activation, C4 deposition, and their contribution to thepathogenesis of antibodymediated rejection. Transplant Rev 2009; 23: 139-50.

[2]   Capra NF. Mechanisms of oral sensation. Dysphagia 1995; 10: 235-47.

[3]   Clark FJ, Horch KW. Kinesthesia. In: Boff KR *et al*, Eds. Handbook of perception and human performance, vol.1 Sensory processes and perception, New York, John Wiley, 1986.

[4]   Linden RWA. Periodontal mechanoreceptors and their function. In Taylor A, Ed. Neurophysiology of the jaws and teeth, Basingstoke,Macmillan, 1990.

[5]   Bligh J, Voigt K. Thermoreception and temperature regulation. Berlin, Springer-Verlag, 1990.

[6]   Spray DC. Cutaneous temperature receptors. Annual review of Physiology 1986; 48:62538.

[7]   van Willigen JD, Schaafsma A, Broekhuijsen MI, Juch PJ. Perception of forces exerted by jaw and thumb. Arch.Oral Biol. 1992; 37:779 88

[8]   Boyd IA, Gladden KW, Eds. The muscle spindle. New York, Stockton press, 1985.

[9]   Capra NF, Ro JY, Wax TD. Physiological identification of jaw-movement-related neurons in the trigeminal nucleus of cats. Somatosens Mot .Res 2002; 11:77 88.

[10]   Radovanovic S, Korotkov A, Ljubisavlievic M *et al*. Comparison of brain activity during different types of proprioceptive inputs: a positron emission tomography study. Exp Brain Res. 2002 ; 143:276 85.

[11]   Norgren R. The Gustatory System. In: The Human Nervous System. Paxinos G, Eds, Academic Press, 1990.

[12]   Gilbertson TA, Damak S, Margolskee RF. The Molecular Physiology of Taste Transduction. Current Opinion in Neurobiology, 2000; 10:519-27.

[13]   Garrett JR. The proper role of nerves in salivary secretion: a review. Journal of Dental Research 1987; 66:387.

[14]   Smith DV, John S.J.St. Neural Coding of Gustatory Information. Current Opinion in Neurobiology 1999; 9:427-35.

[15]   Wayler AH, Perlmuter LC, Cardello AV et al. Effects of age and removable artificial dentition on taste. Spec Care Dentist 1990; 10: 107-13.

[16]   Kinnamon SC. Taste transduction: diversity of mechanisms. Trends in Neuroscience 1988; 11:491 6.

[17]   Mott AE, Leopold DA. Disorders in taste and smell. Medical Clinics of

[18]   North America 1991; 75:1321 53.

[19]   Pedersen AM, Bardow A, Jensen SB, Nauntofte B. Saliva and gastrointestinal functions on taste, mastication, swallowing and digestion. Oral diseases 2002; 8:117 29.

[20]   Baum BJ. Principles of saliva secretion. Ann NY Acad Sci 1993; 694:17 23.

[21]   Won S, Kho H, Kim Y *et al*. Analysis of residual saliva and minor

[22]   salivary gland secretions. Arch Oral Biol. 2001; 46: 619-24.

[23]   21.van Nieuw Amerongen A. The functions of saliva. Ned Tijdschr Tandheelkd 1992; 99: 78-81.

CHAPTER 4

Oral Microbial Flora

Anastasios K. Markopoulos

Aristotle University of Thessaloniki

Abstract: The normal oral flora of humans is exceedingly complex and consists of more than 200 species of bacteria. The composition of the oral flora may be influenced by various factors, including oral hygiene, genetics, age, sex, stress and diet of the individual. At birth, the mucous membranes of the mouth and pharynx are often sterile at birth but may be contaminated by passage through the birth canal 4-12 hours after birth. The development of the teeth is accompanied by the appearance of other regions, which may provide suitable conditions for growth of microorganisms.

COMPOSITION OF ORAL MICROBIAL FLORA

bacteria

fungi

mycoplasms

viruses

protozoa

More than 200 bacterial species have been isolated by the flora of mouth. However the permanent oral flora is composed of 20 bacterial types.

Oral microbial flora consists of:

Gram-positive cocci

Gram-negative cocci

Gram-positive bacteria

Gram-negative bacteria

Gram-positive cocci are:

Streptococci

- S.mutans
- S.sanguis
- S.mitis
- S.milleri
- S.salivarius

S.mutans

- primary cause of caries
- it has the capability to synthesize polysaccharides
- it produces mutacines contributing to the ecological environment configuration in microbial plaque

S.sanguis

- selectively colonizes the surfaces of teeth
- it has the capacity to synthesize polysaccharides
- it is found in the endocardium of individuals suffering from endocarditis

S.mitis

- colonizes the surfaces of teeth
- it is usually found in cases of bacteremia after tooth extraction
- it is found in the endocardium of individuals suffering from endocarditis

S.milleri

- it was isolated for first time from pus of dental abscesses
- it is found in the flora of gingival crevice.

S.salivarius

- selectively colonizes the mucosal surfaces (mainly the tongue)
- it is found in saliva

Staphylococci

- in the oral environment they are found in low percentage proportions
- mainly *S.aureus* (50%)

Gram-negative cocci are:

- *Neisseriae*
- *Veillonellae*

Neisseriae

- they are usually found on dental or mucosal surfaces
- they metabolize lactic acid

Veillonellae

- they metabolize lactic acid
- probably they block the formation of tooth decay

Gram-positive bacteria

- *actinomyces*
- *lactobacilli*
- *corynobacteria*

Actinomyces

- bovis, israelii, naeslundi, viscosous
- they contribute in the creation and maturation of microbial plaque
- they are attached with other bacteria

Lactobacilli

- they are mainly found in the palate
- they have carious action

<u>Gram-negative bacteria</u>

- *bacteroides*
- *fusobacteria*
- *capnocytophaga*
- *actinobacilli*
- *speirochetes*

Bacteroides

Bacteroides melaninogenicus

- *B.gingivalis*
- *B.intermedius*

Bacteroides gingivalis

- it causes formation of abscesses
- it inhibits chemiotaxis of polymorphonuclear cells
- it decreases the phagocytosis
- it resists to the action of supplement

Bacteroides intermedius

- causes formation of abscesses (in smaller degree than *B. gingivalis*)

Fusobacteria

- *Fusobacterium nucleatum*
- *Fusobacterium periodonticum*
- they are involved in various infections in collaboration with speirochetes

Capnocytophaga

- *gingivalis, ochracea, sputigena*
- they are found in the palate and in the gingival crevice
- inhibit chemiotaxis of polymorphonuclear cells

Actinobacilli

- *A. actinomycetemcomitans*
- they inhibit chemiotaxis of polymorphonuclear cells
- they alter the operations of lymphocytes
- they are detected in 90% of individuals suffering from juvenile periodontitis

Speirochetes

- *Treponema denticola*
- *Treponema orale*
- *Treponema macrodentica*
- they are located in the flora of gingival crevice

Fungi

- Their presence is depended from pH the oral cavity
- *Candida albicans*
- *Candida krusei*

Other microorganisms

- - Viruses: *Herpes simple virus* (HSV)
- - *Mycoplasms: Mycoplasma oralis*
- - Protozoa: *Entamoeba gingivalis, Trichomonas tenax*

Effect of Oral Flora in the Host

The effect of oral flora in the host is both beneficial and malicious.

Beneficial effects

■ Microorganisms produce substances used by the host for its metabolic needs (i.e. vitamins B and K)

■ Due to the competition between saprophytic and pathogenic microorganisms there is no activity of pathogenic microorganisma

■ Host's natural immunity is increased

■ Malicious effects

■ Dental caries

■ Periodontitis

■ Candidiasis

Distribution of Normal Flora in the Surfaces of Mouth

Due to the different ecological conditions in the oral cavity, the quantitative and qualitative composition of oral flora differs from region to region.

Saliva

➢ Strep. salivarius

➢ Strep. Mitis

➢ Veillonellae

Tongue

Approximately 100 bacteria colonize every epithelial cell of the tongue

➢ Strep. salivarius

➢ Strep. mitis

➢ Staphylococcus

➢ Bacteroides

Buccal/palatal mucosa

~ 5-15 bacteria colonize every epithelial cell

➢ Strep. mitis

Gingival crevice

✓ In this region there is the highest number of bacteria (10^{12} per cm^2)

✓ Mainly they are anaerobe bacteria

- *bacteroides melaninogenicus*

- *speirochetes*

✓ Ratio of anaerobes / aerobes =10/1

Microbial dental plaque

❖ Dental plaque is a soft deposit that forms on the surface of teeth. It contains many types of bacteria

❖ It is a biologic entity that morphologically transforms

❖ Qualitative and quantitative alterations occur in the composition of dental plaque

The alterations of dental plaque depend on:

❑ time

❑ individual

❑ tooth surface morphology

❑ tooth surface region

- supragingival

- subgingival

Dental plaque is an acquired biofilm. Its formation starts with the precipitation of organic substances from saliva. Approximately 100 bacteria per cm^2 are attached on the initial dental plaque.

The main bacteria in dental plaque are:

- Strep. Sanguis

- Actinomyces

- Lactobacilli

After 1-2 days, the number of attached bacteria increases to 107-108 bacteria /cm^2. Now the main bacteria are:

✓ Strep. sanguis

✓ Anaerobic bacteria

✓ Veillonellae

✓ Peptostreptococci

While the initial dental plaque mainly contains aerobic bacteria, in the mature dental plaque there is a predominance of anaerobic bacteria.

The arrangement of bacteria in dental plaque may be:

➢ colonial

➢ heterogenous

Heterogenous type is usually found in deeper layers of dental plaque.

Dental calculus is the calcified mature dental plaque. Formation of supragingival dental calculus is related with microorganisms of the dental plaque, while the formation of subgingival with white cells.

The most common microorganisms of dental plaque are:

✓ Streptococci

✓ Actinomyces

✓ Gram negative bacteria

  - *leptotrichia buccalis*

  - *bacteroides*

Factors affecting the composition of oral flora are:

✓ Temperature

✓ pH

✓ nutritional substances

✓ anaerobiosis

✓ swallowing movements

✓ antimicrobial factors

✓ microorganism interactions

✓ age

Temperature

✓ directly affects microbial metabolism

✓ indirectly affects pH, ionic power and enzymic activity

pH

✓ most microorganisms are not acidophilic and require a pH of 6.5 - 7.5

✓ acidophilic are also some *streptococci*, *lactobacilli* and *fungi*

✓ Salivary pH affects mucosal and hard tissues pH

Anaerobiosis

Despite the fact that oral cavity is rich in oxygen, there are regions where anaerobic conditions dominate. These regions are

✓ gingival crevice

✓ interproximal spaces of teeth

✓ alveolar vestibules

✓ mature dental plaque

Swallowing movements

■ During the daytime approximately 590 swallowing movements are performed. During the night their number falls to 50

■ At the intervals between meals, bacterial flora is increased

Nutritional substances

The presence or not of the nutritional substances determines the phenotypic expression of microorganisms

■ sheath synthesis

■ susceptibility to antibiotics

- ■ enzymic activity

- ■ polysaccharides production

Antimicrobial agents

- ➤ lactoferrin

- ➤ lysozyme

- ➤ lactoperoxidase system

- ➤ immunoglobulins

- ➤ complement

- ➤ salivary isohaemagglutinins

- ➤ white cells

Microbial interactions

Competitive or accessory interactions may be developed between different microorganisms. This favors or may lead to the inhibition of the development of one of the microorganisms.

Age

- ■ The oral cavity of neonates is sterile of bacteria

- ■ Bacterial colonization begins 6-10 hours after the delivery

- ■ During the first days of life the presence of *Strep.*salivarius is approximately 98%

- ■ During the first days of life aerobic microorganisms prevail. However gradually as teeth erupt the numer of anaerobes is significantly increased

The oral microbial flora in children and adults is almost identical

Exemptions are:

- ✓ speirochetes

- ✓ bacteroides melaninogenicus

- ✓ actinomyces viscosus

Those settle in oral flora after the age of 12-14 years [1-9]

BIOFILMS

Definition of Biofilm

Organized aggregation of bacterial populations, which are surrounded by organic matrix and remain attached to the surfaces. Several studies have shown that the participating bacteria in an oral biofilm differ genetically from those who develop isolated. Close adjacency of bacteria in biofilms gives them the capacity of quorum sensing due to exchange of chemical messages.

Common Characteristics of Biofilms

- ✓ Bacterial presence

- ✓ Presence of extracellular matrix produced by bacteria

- ✓ Stable surface

Modified Definition of Biofilms

An organized bacterial community composed of cells whose characteristics are:

✓ Irreversible attachment on surfaces or matrix

✓ Incorporation in extracellular organic matrix

✓ Development of differentiated phenotype as regards the genetic expression

Studies with confocal scanning microscope showed that:

✓ Biofilms rather develop as microcolonies and not as homogeneous coatings

✓ Numerous bacterial strains are usually participating in biofilms

✓ 15% of the biofilm mass are bacteria, while the remaining 85% extracellular matrix

✓ Between the bacterial microcolonies there is a network of water channels

Tractive Forces for Biofilm Formation

✓ Van der Waals forces. They are weak, 1kcal/mole, 3-4 A, or >50nm)

✓ Electrostatic forces. They are stronger , 10-20 nm, 3-7 kcal/mole, in dry environment

✓ H2-bond reactions. They usually occur between proteins, 3-7 kcal/mole

✓ Hydrophobic or hydrophilic reactions. They are a combination of H2-bond and electrostatic reactions and usually are effective in distances less than 1.5 nm

Van der Waals forces are responsible for the formation of oral biofilms on the surfaces of the oral cavity

Biofilm Formation on the Surfaces of the Oral Cavity

✓ Negative and positive ions on the surface (PO_4 and Ca^{++}) attract bigger molecules (i.e. glycoproteins)

✓ Usually, binding takes place directly

✓ Enamel pellicle is the accumulation of glycoproteins on enamel surface

✓ Glycoproteins having COO-, SO_4 and OH- roots are the most frequently attached substances on dental surfaces

✓ Glycoproteins may also bind with enamel's NH+ roots

✓ Enamel's surface is amphoteric

Salivary constituents having the biggest tendency binding with enamel are proteins containing:

✓ Cysteine

✓ Histidine

✓ Tyrosine

Salivary constituents having the biggest tendency binding with enamel are proteins containing:

✓ Tryptophane

✓ Phenylalanine

✓ Proline

BACTERIAL ADHERENCE ON THE ORAL SURFACES

The marginal thickness of biofilms permitting bacterial adherence is 30-40μ. Below this thickness, bacterial adherence is impossible.

Bacterial adherence on the oral surfaces takes place into three phases:

➢ the first two phases are reversible and depend on hydrophobic reactions

➢ the third is irreversible and depends on bacterial metabolic products (glycans or dextrans) which act as a "biologic glue".

Tractive Forces for Bacterial Adherence in the First Two Phases

- Van der Waals forces (when distance is>50 nm)

- Van der Waals and electrostatic forces (when distance = 10-20 nm)

- hydrophobic, electrostatic and lectin (when distance is <1.5 nm)

These tractive forces are depended on the bacterial ability to remove H_2O from the local environment.

Tractive Forces for Bacterial Adherence in the Third Phase

- ✓ electrostatic reactions

- ✓ lectin reactions

Electrostatic Reactions

They are forces developed between the negatively charged bacteria and glycoproteins of the acquired pellicle. Most microorganisms are negatively charged. An important factor contributing to the creation of negative bacterial forces is the presence of teichoic acids in the bacterial cell wall.

Lectin Reactions

Reactions of bacterial carbohydrates with regions of the acquired pellicle containing lectins.

Factors Contributing to Bacterial Adherence

- ➢ gluteous coating

- ➢ pili

- ➢ streptococcal protein M and teichoic acids

- ➢ β2 microglobulins

Gluteous coating: Surrounds the bodies of certain bacteria. It is probably composed of polysaccharides.

- ✓ s.mutans, s.salivarius

- ✓ A.naeslundi, A.viscosus, A.israeli

- ✓ A.actinomycetemcomitans

- ✓ capnocytophaga

Pili: Small fibrillar projections of the cell membrane of certain bacteria.

Streptococcal protein M and teichoic acids: Protein M is mainly found in the external streptococcal wall. Teichoic acids are attached on specific receptors found on epithelial cells.

β2 microglobulins: They are found in small quantities on the cytoplasmic membrane of cells and probably represent targets of certain streptococcal species

How Fluorides Influence Biofilm Formation

- They have competitive action with other ions in the binding sites

- They alter the charges of dental surfaces making bacterial adherence impossible

How Chlorexidine Affects Pellicle Formation

- It is bacteriostatic

- It reduces negative charges of dental surfaces

BACTERIAL METABOLISM

Bacteria have a complex enzymatic system whose main goal is to retrieve energy from other substances.

Bacterial Metabolic Ways

■ oxidative phosphorylization

■ glycolysis

Certain bacteria use oxidative phosphorylization in order to produce ATP. They metabolize carbohydrates or proteins and finally retrieve energy from Krebs cycle. Krebs cycle requires O_2. However, most bacteria of the oral cavity use glycolysis to produce ATP. Glycolysis leads to the production of lactic acid.

Bacterial Metabolism Starts:

✓ at the extracellular bacterial environment

✓ at the bacterial body

Most Bacteria Prefer Sucrose for their Metabolism Because:

✓ it provides high levels of energy

✓ certain sucrose products (dextranes) contribute to the bacterial attachment

In the Extracellular Environment Sucrose Begins to Catabolize into:

➢ glucose

➢ fructose

➢ soluble or insoluble polysaccharides

The intracellular metabolism of carbohydrates begins after the entrance of monosaccharides in the bacterial body

Factors Affecting Bacterial Carious Action

✓ lactic acid production

✓ glycans action

The action of lactic acid itself is not enough for dental caries formation. Formation of dental caries prerequisites lactic acid action in a localized and special configured environment. This special environment is configured by glycans.

ENZYMATIC SYSTEMS USED IN BACTERIAL METABOLISM

✓ Enzymes play a significant role in the biologic systems

✓ They are chemical substances having the capacity of altering certain characteristics of a chemical

✓ Almost every chemical reaction in human organism is assisted by enzymes

An example of enzymatic action is a common chemical reaction of the human body which is catalyzed by the enzyme carbonic dehydrase

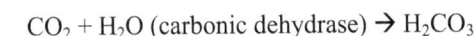

$CO_2 + H_2O$ (carbonic dehydrase) $\rightarrow H_2CO_3$

❖ amount of H_2CO_3 without enzymatic assistance: 10^2 mol/sec

❖ amount of H_2CO_3 with enzymatic assistance: 10^7 mol/sec

Enzymatic Systems Used in Carbohydrates Metabolism

◆ Extracellular invertase systems (km=1-10 nm)

◆ Extracellular glycanes system (km=1-3 nm)

◆ Transferases system

Extracellular invertase systems

✓   This system catalyzes the reaction sucrose (invertase) → fructose + glucose

Extracellular glycans system (glycosyltransferases)

✓   This system catalyzes the reaction sucrose → dextrans + glycans and participates in dental caries

Transferases systems

♦   transferases system is the most complex from all three enzymatic systems

♦   in a first phase glucose is phosphorylated in a second phase glucose is transferred through cell membrane

REFERENCES

[1]   Ali RW, Velcescu C, Jivanescu MC, Lofthus B, Skaug N. Prevalence of 6 putative periodontal pathogens in subgingival plaque samples from Romanian adult periodontitis patients. J Clin Periodontol 1996; 23:133-139

[2]   Haukioja A, Ihalin R, Loimaranta V, Lenander M, Tenovuo, J. Sensitivity of Helicobacter pylori to an innate defence mechanism, the lactoperoxidase system, in buffer and in human whole saliva. J Med Microbiol 2004; 53: 855-860

[3]   Hellström MK, Ramberg P, Krok L, Lindhe J. The effect of supragingival plaque control on the subgingival microflora in human periodontitis. J Clin Periodontol 1996; 23: 934-940

[4]   Ihalin R, Loimaranta V, Tenovuo J. Origin, structure, and biological activities of peroxidases in human saliva. Arch Biochem Biophys 2006; 445: 261-268

[5]   Ihalin R, Pienihäkkinen K, Lenander M, Tenovuo J, Jousimies-Somer H. Susceptibilities of different Actinobacillus actinomycetemcomitans strains to lactoperoxidase-iodide-hydrogen peroxide combination and different antibiotics. Int. J. Antimicrob. Agents 2003; 21: 434-440

[6]   Papapanou PN, Madianos PN, Dahlen G, Sandros J. "Checkerboard" versus culture: a comparison between two methods for identification of subgingival microbiota. Eur J Oral Sci. 1997; 105: 389-396

[7]   Roberts A. Bacteria in the mouth. Dent Update 2005; 32: 134-136

[8]   Tenovuo J. Antimicrobial agents in saliva – protection for the whole body. J. Dent. Res. 2002;81: 807-809

[9]   Välimaa H, Waris M., Hukkanen V, Blankenvoorde M.FJ, Amerongen AV, Tenovuo J. Salivary defence factors in herpes simplex virus infection. J. Dent. Res. 2002; 81: 416- 421

CHAPTER 5

Mastication

Anastasios K.Markopoulos

Aristotle University of Thessaloniki

Abstract: Mastication is the first stage in the process of digestion. In most mammals, controlled vertical and transverse movements of the mandible, as well as protrusion and retrusion of the tongue characterize mastication.

These controlled movements of the mandible contribute also in swallowing and production of speech. In these functions significant is also the contribution of tongue and certain muscles controlling perioral area, pharynx and larynx.

The controlled movements of mastication are not observed from the initial stages of life. However, some non-synchronized movements of mandible start from embryonic life in all mammals. During neonatal life, several masticatory movements are observed, but most mammals are feeded with sucking. Later a gradual shift of kinetic prototypes of sucking to the prototypes of mastication occurs. Mechanisms controlling this shift are multifactorial and are probably related with maturation of neural and anatomic components.

MOVEMENTS OF MASTICATION

During mastication, mouth opens and closes with rhythmical movements. The type of mandible movements differs from mammal to mammal and depends on the type of the food. Despite the discrepancies between different mammal species, we could subdivide masticatory cycle into four phases. The first phase is characterized by a slow opening of the mandible. In the second phase, the opening becomes faster. During the third phase, a rapid closing is observed. In the fourth phase (occlusal or intercuspal) there is a deceleration of the closing speed, which results in food crushing between teeth. Numerous techniques have been proposed for masticatory cycle movements tracing. The most significant are cinephotography, cinefluorography, movement analysis with electronic computer and use of high speed camera recording certain points of reference. Masticatory process is composed of repetitive masticatory cycles starting with food intake and ending with swallowing. This process can be subdivided into three periods. During the first period, the food is chopped and is transferred to the posterior teeth. At the second period, bolus is formed and the third period is characterized as period before swallowing [1]. During mastication, tongue plays a significant role in food transfer and in bolus formation. Solid and liquid foods are transferred through the oral cavity with tongue's help. During the initial phase of masticatory cycle, tongue is moved anteriorly in order to receive the incoming food. During second and third phase with the help of hyoid bone, food is transferred posteriorly. After mastication, tongue significantly contributes in bolus transfer beyond soft palate. Another function performed by tongue is the return of food not adequately crushed and shrinked [2].

Muscle Activity During Mastication

The type of muscle activity controlling the movements of mandible depends on several factors. Most important are the mammal species and the hardness of the food.

Jaw opening muscles remain inactive during the closure of mandible. In contrast, jaw closing muscles are active during that period. Activation of jaw opening muscles is observed during jaw opening. Contraction of jaw opening muscles is intensified at that time when food is crushed between teeth. The side in which crushing of food is performed is termed working side [3]. The degree of contraction of jaw opening muscles is significantly higher in working side compared with non-working side [4].

What is Electromyogram

Cellular unit in a muscle is the muscle cell or muscular fiber. Muscular fiber is connected with an a-kinetic neuron. Alpha-neuron, abductory fiber and all muscular fibers are termed motor unit. Activation of a-kinetic neuron results in the contraction of muscle fibers. During the muscular contraction alterations in the electrical charges of muscle fibers occur. These alterations can be recorded with the use of appropriate electrodes placed on the surface of the muscle. The sum of the recorded alterations is called electromyogram. The rate of the electrical charges significantly depends on the size and the number of the kinetic units. It is also influenced from the location and the type of the recording electrodes [5-7].

As for the type of electrodes, there are three main categories;

✓ isolated surface electrodes

✓ multiple surface electrodes

✓ implanted electrodes

Isolated electrodes record the activity of isolated muscles. Multiple electrodes record the activity of muscle groups, while implanted electrodes are used when muscles are not accessible to surface electrodes.

Despite certain limitations, electromyogram provides significant information regarding jaw opening and closing muscles condition. Its validity is significantly increased when it is combined with the recording of jaw movements.

5.2 BRAINSTEM CONTROL OF MASTICATION

Brainstem is the lower part of the brain, adjoining and structurally continuous with the spinal cord. The brainstem provides the main motor and sensory innervations to the face and neck via the cranial nerves. It is an extremely important region as several nerve connections of the motor and sensory systems of the brain pass through the brainstem.

Brainstem

Brainstem significantly helps for the final regulation of several homeostatic functions. It represents a basic tool for the organism's survival.

In every mammal, brainstem is composed out of three regions;

✓ medulla oblongata (myelencephalon)

✓ pons varoli (metencephalon) and

✓ the biggest part of midbrain (mesencephalon)

These three regions contain several nuclei of important neurons called cranial nerves. Totally, there are twelve pairs of cranial nerves (Table 1).

Table 1: Cranial Nerves

	Name of nerve	**Nuclei**	**Target**
I	Olfactory	Anterior olfactory nucleus	Olfactory mucosa
II	Optic	Lateral geniculate nucleus	Retina
III	Oculomotor nerve	Oculomotor nucleus	-Ocular muscles -Upper eyelid muscles
IV	Trochlear	Trochlear nucleus	Superior oblique ophthalmic muscle
V	Trigeminal	Principal sensory trigeminal nucleus, Spinal trigeminal nucleus, Mesencephalic trigeminal nucleus, Trigeminal motor nucleus	-Ocular region -Maxilla -Mandible -Tongue

Table 2 cont....

VI	Abducens nerve	Abducens nucleus	Lateral rectus, which abducts the eye
VII	Facial	Facial nucleus, Solitary nucleus, Superior salivatory nucleus	Provides motor innervation to the muscles of facial expression and stapedius, receives the sense of taste from the anterior 2/3 of the tongue, and provides secretomotor innervation to the salivary glands (except parotid) and the lacrimal gland
VIII	Vestibulocochlear nerve	Lateral to cranial nerve VII	-Neuroepithelial cells of Corti apparatus, Vestibular nuclei, Cochlear nuclei
IX	Glossopharyngeal	Medulla oblongata	provides secretomotor innervation to the parotid gland, provides motor innervation to the stylopharyngeus muscle, innervates the posterior region of tongue and taste bud mucosa
X	Vagus	Mixed nucleus of medulla oblongata	-Striped laryngeal and pharyngeal muscles -Skin of external acoustic duct -Pharyngeal and laryngeal mucosa -Thoracic and abdominal internal organs
XI	Accessory nerve	- Mixed nucleus of medulla oblongata -Anterior A1,A5 neurotome horns	-Striped pharyngeal and laryngeal muscles -Sternocleidomastoid and trapezoid muscle
XII	Hypoglossal	Medulla oblongata	Muscles of tongue

In brainstem there are also important nuclei not related with cranial nerves. Brainstem possesses a significant degree of autonomy in its functions. However, in certain occasions it is controlled by higher cerebral centers. It is also interconnected with spinal cord. Table 2 illustrates the brainstem regions and the cranial nerves that every region contains.

Table 2: Brainstem regions and their relation with cranial nerves

Brainstem region	**Cranial nerves**
Midbrain	Oculomotor nerve Trochlear
Pons varoli	Trigeminal Abducens Facial Acoustic
Medulla oblongata	Glossopharyngeal Vagus Accessory nerve Hypoglossal

All mandible movements require a combined effort of all masticatory muscles. The whole process is controlled by trigeminal, hypoglossal, facial and other kinetic brainstem nuclei [8-12]. Coordination of these nuclei depends on the abductory impulses from oral cavity, which end to the trigeminal and solitary tract nucleus.

Trigeminal Sensory Nucleus

Trigeminal sensory nucleus consists of a bundle of neurons extending from brainstem to the spinal cord. The rostral region of the nucleus is termed primary sensory nucleus, while the remaininig trigeminal spinal nucleus. Trigeminal spinal nucleus is further subdivided into nucleus oralis, interpolaris and nucleus caudalis.

The central parts of trigeminal sensory nucleus are ramified into ascending or descending branches or they enter into brainstem where they form the trigeminal bundle.

The anterior region of trigeminal pack relates with primary sensory nucleus, while the caudal forms the trigeminal spinal bundle.

Trigeminal sensory nucleus consists of various neurons categories:

✓ local circuit neurons

✓ neurons extending to the brainstem

✓ neurons useful for interconnections inside trigeminal sensory nucleus

Primary sensory nucleus is located on the level of the trigeminal kinetic nucleus.

It is characterized by the lack of dense neuronal bundles and by the lack of large neurons with elongated dendritic projections. Neurons of trigeminal sensory nucleus are responsible for the innervation of rostral and ventral face.

Trigeminal Mesencephalic Nucleus

Trigeminal mesencephalic axis mainly consists of the cellular bodies of the mechanoreceptors of jaw opening muscles, periodontal ligament, gingival and palate.

Neurons of trigeminal mesencephalic nucleus are unipolar and consist of central and peripheral branches. Central branches are heading towards trigeminal kinetic nucleus, while peripheral branches towards the oral cavity regions.

Trigeminal Kinetic Nucleus

Trigeminal kinetic nucleus is composed of neurons controlling the masticatory muscles. These neurons consist of γ and α-kinetic neurons. Kinetic neurons responsible for control of jaw opening muscles are found in the dorsal surface of trigeminal kinetic nucleus, while the neurons responsible for jaw closing muscles are located in the ventral surface of the nucleus.

Hypoglossal Kinetic Nucleus

Hypoglossal kinetic nucleus controls the muscles of the tongue. Structurally, it is more homogeneous compared with trigeminal kinetic nucleus. It consists of large multipolar kinetic neurons and of smaller intermediate neurons. The elongated dendritic projections of kinetic neurons may enter into the adjacent reticular formation.

Facial Kinetic Nucleus

Facial kinetic nucleus is composed of three elongated columns of kinetic neurons; lateral, medial and intermediate separating the first two.

Muscles controlling upper lip, nostrils and nasal cavities are related with neurons of the lateral column of facial kinetic nucleus. The muscular system of lower lip is controlled by kinetic neurons of the intermediate column.

Kinetic neurons of the medial column control other facial and aural regions.

Control of Mastication

Sensory and kinetic brainstem nuclei play a significant role in mastication control.

Today it is believed that the rhythmical masticatory movements of the mandible are generated in a certain brainstem region. Masticatory function is then regulated by afferent sensory impulses to the brainstem nuclei. Synchronization of the whole process is performed by the higher cerebral centers.

Brainstem Activity

Certain brainstem neuronal circuits form a neural network having the capacity to generate rhythmical masticatory movements of the mandible. This network has been termed chewing pattern generator or masticatory center.

Brainstem possesses similar generators responsible for swallowing and respiratory function. However, the precise location of these generators has not yet been clarified.

Significant step towards the understanding of brainstem activity in mastication is the study of various masticatory reflexes.

Masticatory reflexes are subdivided in:

- ✓ reflexes of jaw opening and closing muscles
- ✓ tongue reflexes
- ✓ facial reflexes

Reflexes of the Jaw Opening and Closing Muscles

Jaw reflexes include muscular contractions moving the mandible vertically (opening, closing), horizontally or protrusively-retrusively. Jaw opening and closing muscles include masseters, temporal muscles, lateral and medial pterygoids and digastor. In these muscles, there is a rich network of kinetic neurons extending from trigeminal kinetic nucleus. Exception is the caudal region of digastor, where kinetic neurons extend from accessory facial nucleus.

Jaw Opening Reflex

Several experimental studies have shown that this reflex can be reproduced monosynaptically, either after stimulation of stretch receptors of the jaw opening muscles or after stimulation of the trigeminal mesencephalic nucleus. Jaw opening reflex can be reproduced after slight beating of the chin. Beating of the chin causes distention and therefore stimulation of jaw opening muscles and their mechanoreceptors, which results in activation of the afferent fibers. Afferent fibers through their monosynaptic connections with α-trigeminal kinetic neurons cause contraction of the jaw opening muscles. Jaw opening reflex can also be reproduced after stimulation of mechanoreceptors located in periodontal tissues, temporomandibular joint, oral mucosa or even the skin. As for periodontal mechanoreceptors, they seem to have a short and latent stimulatory effect on the jaw opening kinetic neurons. Observations on anesthetized gingival revealed that jaw-opening reflex was diminished or absent. These findings suggested that periodontal mechanoreceptors are in close adjacency with teeth and occlusal forces are capable of stimulating jaw-opening muscles.

Jaw Closing Reflex

Jaw closing reflex can be produced after mechanical stimulation of periodontal ligament or oral mucosa mechanoreceptors. It is not a monosynaptic reflex. It can also be reproduced after stimulation of other cranial nerves.

Reflexes of Hypoglossal Kinetic Nucleus

This reflex is produced after stimulation of tongue or laryngeal receptors

Facial Reflexes

The reflex of opening and closing of eyelids is produced after stimulation of corneal receptors that are innervated by branches of trigeminal nerve.

Afferent Sensory Impulses to Brainstem Nuclei

Type and texture of food determine the type of masticatory movements. This is achieved through sensory feedback at the brainstem masticatory center. It has been observed that stimulation of different regions of the oral cavity produces different types of masticatory movements. The role of afferent fibers in brainstem masticatory center has been extensively studied. Several studies have shown that immediately after the initiation of mastication, a rhythmical production of electrical charges is observed in the receptors of the jaw opening muscles. Abrupt increase of electrical charges is observed in the beginning and in the end of jaw opening. As for the mechanoreceptors of periodontal ligament, an abrupt increase of electrical charges is observed by the time that teeth come into contact and continue as long as occlusal forces are increased. Abrupt increase of electrical charges is also observed in mechanoreceptors of the corner of the mouth. The fact that electrical charges are low in the other phase of masticatory cycle suggests that tissue distention is the element that stimulates mechanoreceptors.

Synchronization of Masticatory Movements by Higher Cerebral Centers

Electrical stimulation of the lateral part in the kinetic region of brain cortex results in the production of rhythmical repetitive movements of mandible and tongue.

Despite the fact that there is no direct connection between brain cortex and trigeminal kinetic nucleus, electrical stimulation of brain cortex causes short-termed alterations in the jaw closing muscles and low excitativeness in the jaw opening kinetic neurons. These observations lead to the conclusion that higher cerebral centers assist the initiation of masticatory process.

Moreover, electrical stimulation of brain cortex causes movements of the tongue and other orofacial regions. Based on this finding it has been proposed that brain cortex synchronizes the activity of muscular groups involved in masticatory process.

REFERENCES

[1] Amemiya K, Hisano M, Ishida T, Soma K. Relationship between the flow of bolus and occlusal condition during mastication - computer simulation based on the measurement of characteristics of the bolus. J Oral Rehabil 2002; 29:245-56.

[2] Kimoto K, Tamaki K, Toyoda M, Celar AG. Correlation between elevator muscle activity and direction of sagittal closing pathway during unilateral chewing. J Oral Rehabil 2002; 29:430-4.

[3] Bodin C, Lodetti G, Marinone MG. Temporo-mandibular joint kinetics and chewing cycles in children. A 3-year follow-up. Int J Paediatr Dent 2002; 12:33-8.

[4] Bradley RM. Essentials of oral physiology. St Louis, Mosby, 1995, p.p.187-212.

[5] Kobayashi M, Masuda Y, Fujimoto Y *et al.* Electrophysiological analysis of rhythmic jaw movements in the freely moving mouse. Physiol Behav 2002; 75:377-85.

[6] Palomari ET, Vitti M, Tosello Dde et al. Electromyographic study of the masseter muscle in individuals with Class II malocclusion. Electromyogr Clin Neurophysiol 2002; 42: 71-7.

[7] Taylor A. Neurophysiology of the jaws and teeth. Basingstoke, Macmillan, 1990

[8] Dubner R, Sessle BJ, Storey AT. The neural basis of oral and facial function, New York, Plenum press, 1978.

[9] Ishikawa T. Brain regions activated during the mandibular movement tasks in functional magnetic resonance imaging. Kokubyo Gakkai Zasshi 2002 ; 69 : 39-48.

[10] Lund JP. Mastication and its control by the brainstem. Critical reviews in Oral Biology and Medicine 1991; 2:33-64.

[11]   Luschei L, Goldberg LJ. Neural mechanismsof mandibular control: mastication and voluntary biting. In: Handbook of physiology, section 1, The nervous system. Motor control, part 2. American physiological society, Bethesda, Maryland, 1981, Vol 2, p.p. 1237-74.

[12]   Lund JP, Enomoto S. The generation of mastication by the mammalian central nervous system. In: The neural control of rhythmic movements in vertebrates. Cohen AV, Grillner S, Rossignol S, Eds, New York, John Wiley & Sons, 1988.

[13]   Molina OF, dos Santos J, Mazzetto M *et al*. Oral jaw behaviors in TMD and bruxism: a comparison study by severity of bruxism. Cranio 2001; 19:114-22.

CHAPTER 6

Deglutition

Anastasios K.Markopoulos

Aristotle University of Thessaloniki

Abstract: Deglutition is a reflex process of muscular contractions aiming to forward food, saliva or other substances from the oral cavity to stomach.

Although deglutition can be caused consciously, in most instances it is caused subconsciously.

Frequency of deglutition is one per minute, which means that during day and night more than 1000 swallowing movements may occur. Decrease of swallowing activity occurs during sleep.

Beyond food and saliva transportation, deglutition may be protective in nature. In collaboration with respiratory movements, breath is stopped during deglutition, so the entrance of food into trachea is avoided.

In case of food entrance into trachea, apart from other protective reflexes, activation of deglutition occurs that contributes to the cleaning of airways.

Mechanisms of deglutition are complex processes requiring the collaboration of extended parts of the brainstem, cranial nerves, sensory receptors and muscles. Masticatory process is programmed through neural circuits in brainstem's "masticatory center". If masticatory center is activated for a first time, masticatory process becomes then automatic.

MOVEMENTS OF DEGLUTITION

Deglutition is subdivided into four phases; preparatory, oral, pharyngeal and esophageal. Preparatory phase starts immediately after the last phase of mastication and is characterized by bolus formation.

During oral phase, bolus is forwarded from oral cavity to pharynx. Movements of oral phase involve elevation of the anterior one third of the tongue towards palate with simultaneous movement of tongue base down and anteriorly. This results in hypopharyngeal space broadening.

Soft palate is moving up, glossopalatal sphincter is opened and bolus easily passes. Soft palate encounters posterior pharyngeal wall. Nasopharyngeal sphincter contracts the lateral pharyngeal wall minimizing the danger of food entrance in nasal cavity. Lips encounter teeth in the occlusal position. This contact stabilizes mandible at the same time that hyoid bone and larynx perform various movements.

In several individuals, teeth and lips do not make contact during deglutition. In these people, tongue enters between teeth contributing to occlusal and orthodontic problems development.

In the beginning of pharyngeal phase tongue's posterior one third forwards bolus towards hypopharynx. Further bolus forward is achieved with the contractions of pharyngeal sphincters [1].

During pharyngeal phase, epiglottis moves and closes laryngeal vestibule, eliminating the danger of food entrance in larynx. Epiglottal movement is achieved with elevation of hyoid bone and contraction of thyrohyoid muscles.

Finally, opening of esophageal sphincter occurs and esophageal phase is initiated. Esophageal phase starts when blomus arrives at esophageal sphincter. Peristaltic movements of esophagus start from upper esophageal sphincter and in eight seconds arrive in the lower esophageal sphincter [2].

Oral and pharyngeal phase have a short duration. In contrast, oral phase has duration of 0.5 sec, while pharyngeal phase of 0.7 sec.

Esophageal phase has a longer duration. Liquids need 3 sec to arrive in stomach, while solid food 9 sec.

Propulsive Forces on Bolus

Food transportation throughout oral cavity, pharynx an esophagus is achieved due to the presence of a propulsive wave. This wave is formed from pressures exerted by the tongue, peristaltic movements and contractions of muscles and sphincters [3].

In the beginning of masticatory process, air pressure of the oral cavity and pharynx is equal to atmospheric. When mouth is closed and pharyngeal sphincter is contracted, air pressure from oral cavity to the upper esophageal sphincter gradually increases. Pressure increase is due to tongue movements and muscular contractions. In the following 1 sec, relaxation of the upper esophageal sphincter occurs, permitting food passage to esophagus. Further food propulsion takes place by peristaltic movements of the esophageal wall and by forces exerted from new food entering esophagus. Lower esophageal sphincter opens for 3 sec and food enters in stomach.

Muscle activity During Deglutition

Thirty-one pairs of muscles are participating in the process of deglutition. Muscle activity has been recorded and studied with the use of electromyograms [4].

During preparatory and oral phase median pterygoid, masseter, temporal, labial and buccinator are activated.

Pharyngeal phase is characterized by complex activity of the muscles moving:

✓ hyoid bone (mylohyoid, geniohyoid, thyrohyoid, stylohyoid muscles)

✓ tongue (posterior lingual muscles)

✓ pharynx (palatopharyngeal, styloglossus, median and lower sphincters)

✓ larynx (cricothyroid muscles)

Esophageal phase begins 600-800 msec after the initiation of masticatory process. During this phase, there is a continuous activity of esophageal sphincters.

CONTROL OF DEGLUTITION

Preparatory and oral phase of deglutition are unconscious, while pharyngeal and esophageal are conscious.

Today it is believed that kinetic sequence of the muscles participating in masticatory process is controlled by higher cerebral centers and by brainstem's neurons, which form a masticatory center.

Brainstem's masticatory center

Brainstem's masticatory center consists of three parts:

- adductory part

- central part

- abductory part

Afferent part receives fibers originating from oral cavity, pharynx, larynx and esophagus, which end to trigeminal sensory nucleus and nucleus tractus solitarius. These nuclei are responsible for the initiation of pharyngeal phase of deglutition, mainly activating glossopharyngeal muscles.

Masticatory center's central part consists of several sensory and kinetic nuclei interconnected with a dense neural network.

The abductory part is composed of kinetic neurons originating from ambiguus, facial, trigeminal and hypoglossal nucleus as well as of kinetic neurons ending to spinal cord's cervical region.

Deglutition Control by Higher Cerebral Centers

Electrical stimulation of cerebral cortex or other brain regions (internal capsule, amygdala, hypothalamus, substantia nigrans and mesenchephalic reticular formation) has been found to create swallowing movements [5].

The fact that anenchephalic infants or laboratory animals with their brains surgically removed, manifest deglutitional movements, lead to the conclusion that the action of higher cerebral centers is not mandatory for deglutition.

It has been also shown that regardless of region all neural ways participating in deglutition converge into a region, which is brainstem's masticatory center.

Other Neuromuscular Functions Related to Deglutition

Breast-Feeding

Breast-feeding is a complex process based on the application of negative pressure in oral cavity, which is combined with certain infant's movements aiming to extract from mother's breast.

Milk's outflow is achieved with breast's papilla placement in the infant's mouth and its tight obstruction by infant's lips. Negative pressure exerted by jaw movements force milk to outflow.

Negative pressures occurring in breast-feeding vary from 50-200 mm Hg. The number of sucks occurring in breast-feeding depends on the type of breast's papilla and usually is 40-90 per minute.

Breast-feeding is a phenomenon also occurring during gestation. Embryos have the ability to suck and swallow amniotic fluid in while being in uterus.

This fact implies that programming of these movements is performed before birth. The capacity of the swallowed milk is equal with the capacity of milk received during breast-feeding.

Duration of every deglutition in embryos lasts from 1-9 minutes, while their frequency is 7-20 per 24 hours.

Protective Reflexes of Upper Respiratory Tract

Sneeze, coughing, pharyngeal reflex and the sense of drowning are considered protective reflexes that may reproduced after stimulation of pharyngeal and upper respiratory airways. Breath or cardiovascular alterations, swallowing movements and other autonomic reflexes often accompany them.

Laryngeal protective reflexes are resistant in anesthesia, suffocation and in various suppressive medications of central neural system.

These reflexes are easily reproduced in the upper region of larynx. This fact is averting the entrance of food in the upper respiratory airways.

The main larynx's sensory neuron is upper laryngeal branch of vagus nerve.

Laryngeal mucosa is characterized by the presence of numerous sensory nerve endings, which may have the form of a free nerve ending or they may resemble receptors almost identical with taste buds. These receptors are particularly found in epiglottal region.

Receptors of laryngeal mucosa are subdivided into two main categories:

✓   receptors responding to mechanical stimulation of larynx (mechanoreceptors)

✓   receptors responding to chemical stimulation of larynx (chemoreceptors)

The role of mechanoreceptors is significant in the feedback control of deglutition and in the initiation of respiratory airways protective reflexes [6]. Chemoreceptors respond immediately in certain stimulatory odors.

Vomiting

Nausea and vomiting are biologic protective mechanisms aiming to unload organism by swallowed toxic substances.

Vomiting as a reflex particularly develops in carnivorous mammals that rapidly swallow their food and do not devote time for gustatory evaluation [7].

Despite its protective nature, vomiting may be a manifestation of numerous pathologic conditions.

Regardless of the causative factor, in all cases of vomiting nausea precedes.

Nausea is regarded a psychological experience, which can be accompanied by autonomous reflexes, such as increased salivation, mydriasis, sweating and pallidness.

Vomiting has three stages:

-   stage before depletion

-   stage of depletion

-   stage after depletion

Stage before depletion is characterized by increased salivation, pallidness and visceral alterations, such as tachycardia and laxity of stomach. The duration of this stage fluctuates from some minutes to hours or days, especially in pregnant women or patients subjected to chemotherapy.

Stage of depletion starts with a sense of nausea, which ends to a violent food extrusion. Rhythmical respiratory movements with closed epiglottis characterize nausea.

Additionally, a contraction of diaphragm, celiac and external intercostals muscles occurs, resulting in increase of endoceliac pressure. Upper esophageal sphincter opens in every nausea episode. The reason that there is no vomiting in nausea is that muscles behave differently in nausea and vomiting.

Totally 25 nausea episodes may precede vomiting.

Vomiting follows immediately nausea. The main factor causing food extrusion is the muscular contraction of abdominal and external muscles surrounding stomach.

Vomiting is a reflex programmed in neural circuits and medulla oblongata nuclei. Brainstem's medulla oblongata nuclei are interconnected with certain chemoreceptors in the reticular formation.

Medulla oblongata also borders with cardiovascular and masticatory centers.

Vomiting may be produced by several ways. Vomiting center in medulla oblongata may be stimulated by:

✓   increased endocranial pressure

✓   pain

✓   stomach, intestine and urinary cyst lesions

✓   dilatation or uterus injury

✓   damages of vestibular organs

✓   psychological causes

Substances capable of causing vomiting irritate stomach or intestinal mucosa resulting in stimulation of vagus nerve, which is interconnected with brainstem's medulla oblongata.

REFERENCES

[1]   El Haddad MA, Chao CR, Ma SX, Ross MG. Neuronal NO modulates spontaneous and ANG II-stimulated fetal swallowing behavior in the near-term fetus. Am J Physiol Regul Integr Comp Physiol 2002; 282: R1521-7.

[2]   Kendall KA. Oropharyngeal swallowing variability. Laryngoscope 2002; 112: 547-51

[3]   Kitagawa J, Shingai T, Takahashi Y, Yamada Y. Pharyngeal branch of the glossopharyngeal nerve plays a major role in reflex swallowing from the pharynx. Am J Physiol Regul Integr Comp Physiol 2002; 282: R1342-7.

[4]   Miller AJ. Neurophysiological basis of swallowing. Dysphagia 1986; 1:91-100.

[5]   Miller AJ. The search for the central swallowing pathway: the quest for clarity. Dysphagia 1993; 8:185-94.

[6]   Koufman JA, Aviv JE, Casiano RR, Shaw GY. Laryngopharyngeal reflux : position statement of the comittee on speech, voice, and swallowing disorders of the AmericanAcademy of Otolaryngology-Head and Neck Surgery. Otolaryngol Head Neck Surg 2002; 127: 32-5.

[7]   Kucharczyk J, Stewart DJ, Miller AD. Nausea and vomiting: recent research and clinical advances. CRC Press, 1991, Boca Raton

CHAPTER 7

Speech

Anastasios K. Markopoulos

Aristotle University of Thessaloniki

Abstract: Speech is the most common way of communication between people. As a phenomenon, speech is subdivided into two phases, production and perception of speech. Speech production requires the coordinated action of all anatomic elements of vocal tube. The main theories regarding the activity of speech cerebral theories are two; connection theory and modular theory.

Speech is the most common way of communication between people. In other cases, it is useful for the internal communication of every individual and for the facilitation of processes of thought.

As a phenomenon, speech is subdivided into two phases; production and perception of speech.

During the phase of speech production humans are capable to produce 12-14 and to understand 60 phonetic sounds per second.

In order to communicate successfully via the speech the speaker and the listener must use the same language. The phonetic sounds that are used in every language have their own sounds and symbolic meanings.

All languages are characterized by the same common rules. They consist of phones, which in turn form sentences.

Capability of humans for written language has close relationship with speech. It made possible the storage of precious information that has significantly contributed to human development.

The ability for production and perception of oral speech is acquired and to a lesser degree inborn. It starts during the first phases of neonatal life.

Speech perception at the early stages of life is not based on experience of a certain language but on the ability of distinguishing certain sounds.

This ability is due to the development of speech centers in the cerebral cortex from neonatal life. Speech centers exhibit the typical asymmetry of an adult brain, which means that language experience is not a mandatory element for the development of speech centers.

Later on, usually until the age of five years, children learn without particular help their mother tongue. Learning of mother tongue is performed with mimicry, however in the context of a developed and genetically assigned cerebral neural base.

Many organs developed and designed for other functions co participate in phonation and speech production.

Teeth, jaws, lips and tongue are mainly masticatory organs, while lungs, glottidis vocal folds, soft palate and nasal cavity are parts of the respiratory system.

Since all mammals have these organs, the question is why only humans can speak. A possible explanation may be the development of cerebral centers, which have the ability to independently control organs participating in speech production.

Phones are phonetic sounds forming syllables, words and sentences. Every language is composed of a certain group of phones depicted with graphic symbols, known as letters.

Phonemes are the phones separating the meaning in a certain language. They are the smallest <u>segmental</u> units of sound employed to form meaningful contrasts between utterances. They are a group of slightly different sounds, which are all perceived to have the same function by speakers of a language or dialect.

Phonation

<u>Vocal tube</u>: Human vocal tube is an acoustic tube, 17 cm in length, starting from phonetic folds and ending to lips.

Surface of the transverse cutting of vocal tube depends on the position of lips, tongue, jaws and tensor veli palatine. Tensor veli palatine is a term for soft palate used by speech scientists. With proper movements of soft palate, an additional auxiliary space can be used for speech production. This space is the nasal cavity, which is 12 cm in length and has a volume of 60 cm^3.

<u>Phonetic sounds</u>: Phonetic sounds are produced through the increase of air pressure in the lungs and its violent transit through glottis. Glottis is the opening between vocal cords. Transit of air creates oscillation of vocal cords and broad range vibrations, which stimulate vocal tube and create phonetic sounds.

The vibrated part of vocal cords is approximately 18 mm in length. The area of the transverse surface of glottis opening fluctuates from zero to 20 mm^2. Voice increase or decrease depends on the contraction of muscles controlling vocal folds.

Speech Articulation and Resonance

Immediately after their production from vocal tube, sounds are modified and are transformed into speech with the processes of articulation and resonance.

Speech articulation is the process of phonetic sounds transformation into sounds of speech. For the transaction of speech articulation, combined movements of lips, jaws, tongue, palatal and pharyngeal muscles in coordination with phonation and respiratory movements are required.

Resonance is the process in which sounds of speech are filtered. The final form of speech depends on the volume and shape of nasal and oral cavity.

Alterations of nasal and oral cavity depend on the position of the removable parts of pharynx and oral cavity.

Frequency of human speech occupies a broad region of the auditory spectrum. It extends from 300 to 3000 Hz.

Apart from sounds of speech, humans are capable of producing two additional sorts of sounds; fricative and plosive sounds.

For the production of fricative sounds closing of glottis and air pressure increase is needed, which result in turbulence. Fricative sounds require fine movements of the anatomic elements. Fricative sounds quality easily rebates in individuals wearing oral prosthetic appliances or having occlusal problems.

For the production of plosive sounds, a full closure of vocal tube is needed, which results in air pressure increase.

Production of speech movements also requires sensory information provision from all oral mechanoreceptors and muscle receptors to the cerebral centers.

Sensory information provision is needed for the correction of speech mistakes and for regulation of speech accompanying gestures.

CEREBRAL CENTERS OF SPEECH CONTROL

Speech production requires the coordinated action of all anatomic elements of vocal tube.

Kinetic neurons responsible for respiratory system movements are located in the cervical, thoracic and upper lumbar region of spinal cord.

Neurons controlling glottis movements are located in brainstem's nucleus ambiguous, while neurons controlling the articulation movements are found in the upper thoracic region of spinal cord and in trigeminal, facial, hypoglossal and ambiguous nucleus of brainstem.

The fact that surgical excision of brainstems' trigeminal nucleus region in animals, results to loss of vocal ability, lead to the conclusion that the interchange of neural information between brainstem's nuclei and spinal cord is not enough for speech production. Research was then turn to the search of other cerebral centers that could be responsible for speech production. Studies on aphasia, which is usually caused by head injuries or cerebral stroke and is characterized by loss of ability to speak, played a significant role towards this direction.

Observations revealed that only damages of the left hemisphere caused loss of ability for speech. Further studies showed that two cerebral regions are responsible for speech production; Broca's and Wernicke's centers. These regions adjoin with acoustic cortex and central brain sulcus and as was later confirmed they are also related with capability for notional language.

Unilateral control of cerebral functions in humans by the left-brain hemisphere, definitely suggests a cerebral dominance of the left towards the right-brain hemisphere.

Activity of the Cerebral Speech Centers

Several studies have worked on the issue of speech production and have suggested some theoretical models regarding the activity of speech cerebral centers.

The main theories are two; connection theory and modular theory.

According to connection theory, when human ear listens a word, immediately transfers this information to acoustic cortex in Wernicke's center.

If the person intends to answer to the word, information is transferred from Wernicke's to Broca's center and to cerebral cortex. Information regarding speech articulation is generated in

Broca's center and cerebral cortex and are send in brainstem's kinetic nuclei controlling the responsible for speech muscles.

If the person saw a written word, optical information arrive from optical centers in angular gyrus where they are transformed in auditory, relevant with the word information and are send in Wernicke's center.

In other words, connection theory proposes that language understanding is performed in Wernicke's center and speech production starts with information provision from Wernicke's to Broca's center and to cerebral cortex. Information is then send to brainstem nuclei, which control the responsible muscles for speech production.

Connection theory failed to answer several questions. One question was why cerebral damages after injuries or pathologic conditions in multilingual persons impaired the ability for only one language and not for all.

Another issue not adequately solved by connection theory was the complexicity of speech information. Every language contains different types of information, such as sounds, grammatical information and word meanings.

For the above reasons connection theory was replaced by modular theory.

According to this theory the cerebral region, which is related with speech and language is not homogeneous but is subdivided into multiple units.

Every unit is responsible for a different language.

DISTURBANCES OF SPEECH

The shape of vocal tube plays a significant role in resonance and articulation of speech. If the shape of oral cavity changes, which usually happens in patients with orthodontic or prosthetic appliances, patient has to modify the articulation of his speech. Many patients get through and neuromusculary adjust to the new anatomic condition, while others are having difficulties in speech articulation. Usually full dentures are causing slight speech alterations. However, the majority of patients quickly adjust to the new way of speech.

REFERENCES

[1]   Damasio AR. The neural basis of language. Ann Rev Neurosci 1984; 7:127-47.
[2]   Koufman JA, Aviv JE, Casiano RR, Shaw GY. Laryngopharyngeal reflux: position statement of the committee on speech, voice, and swallowing disorders of the American Academy of Otolaryngology-Head and Neck Surgery. Otolaryngol Head Neck Surg 2002; 127: 32-5.
[3]   Larsen SG, Hudson FG. Oral kinesthetic sensitivity and the perception of speech. Child Dev 1973; 44: 845-8.
[4]   Werker JF, Tees RC. The organization and reorganization of human speech perception. Trends in Neuroscience 1981; 4:135-7.

SUBJECT INDEX

www.ingramcontent.com/pod-product-compliance
Lightning Source LLC
Chambersburg PA
CBHW080021240326
41598CB00075B/750